Study Guide to Accompany

STRUCTURE & FUNCTION OF THE BODY

Eleventh Edition

Prepared by
Linda Swisher, R.N., Ed.D.
Sarasota County Technical Institute
Sarasota, Florida

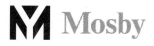
Mosby

An Imprint of Elsevier Science

St. Louis   London   Philadelphia   Sydney   Toronto

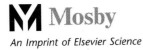
Mosby
An Imprint of Elsevier Science

Vice President, Nursing Editorial Director: Sally Schrefer
Executive Editor: June Thompson
Developmental Editor: Billi Carcheri Sharp
Project Manager: Gayle Morris
Book Designer: Mark Oberkrom

Copyright © 2000 by Mosby, Inc.

Previous editions copyrighted 1997.

Printed in the United States of America

Mosby, Inc.
An Imprint of Elsevier Science
11830 Westline Industrial Drive
St. Louis, Missouri 63146

ISBN: 0-323-01080-6

02 03 04 BD/KPT 9 8 7 6 5

Preface

To the Instructor

This study guide is designed to help your students master basic anatomy and physiology. It works in two ways.

First, the section of the preface titled "To the Student" contains detailed information about the following topics:

- How to achieve good grades in anatomy and physiology

- How to read the textbook

- How to use the exercises in this study guide

- How to use visual memory as a learning tool

- How to use mnemonic devices as learning aids

- How to prepare for an examination

- How to take an examination

- How to find out why questions were missed on an examination

Second, the study guide itself contains features that facilitate learning. These features include the following:

1. LEARNING OBJECTIVES, designed to break down the information to be mastered into smaller, more manageable units. The questions in this study guide have been developed to help the student master the learning objectives that are identified at the beginning of each chapter in the text. The guide is also sequenced to correspond to key areas of each chapter. A variety of questions has been prepared to cover the material effectively and to expose the student to several different approaches to learning.
2. CROSSWORD PUZZLES and WORD FINDS, to encourage the use of new vocabulary words and emphasize the proper spelling of these terms.
3. OPTIONAL APPLICATION QUESTIONS, particularly targeted for the health occupations student but appropriate for any student of anatomy and physiology because they are based entirely on information contained within the chapter.
4. DIAGRAMS, with key features marked by numbers for identification. Students can easily check their work by comparing the diagram in the workbook with the equivalent figure in the text.

5. PAGE NUMBER REFERENCES, found in the "Answers to Chapter Exercises" section. Each answer is cross-referenced with the page in the text where the information supporting that answer is found. Additionally, questions are grouped by specific topics that correspond to sections of the text. Following each major section of the study guide are references to specific areas of the text that will help students who are having difficulty with a particular grouping of questions. These references will point the students to the part of the text on which they should focus their study. These references are of great assistance to both instructor and student because remedial work is made easier and more effective when the area of weakness is identified accurately.

These features should make mastery of the material contained in this text and study guide a rewarding experience for both instructor and student.

To the Student

How to Achieve Good Grades in Anatomy and Physiology

This study guide is designed to help you be successful in learning anatomy and physiology. Before you begin using the study guide, read the following suggestions. Understanding effective study techniques and having good study habits will help you become a more successful student.

How to Read the Textbook

Keep up with the reading assignments. Read the textbook assignment before the instructor covers the material in a lecture. If you have failed to read the assignment beforehand, you will not grasp what the instructor is talking about in lecture. When you read, do the following:

1. As you finish reading a sentence, ask yourself if you understand it. If you do not, put a question mark in the margin by that sentence. If the instructor does not clear up the problem in a lecture, ask him or her to explain it to you.
2. Make sure you can perform all of the learning objectives in the text. A learning objective is a specific task that you are expected to be able to do after you have read a chapter. The objectives set specific goals and break down learning into small steps. They emphasize the key points that the author is making in the chapter.
3. Underline the text and make notes in the margin to highlight key ideas, to mark something you need to reinforce at a later time, or to indicate things that you do not understand.
4. If you come to a word you do not understand, look it up in a dictionary. Write the word on one side of an index card, and write its definition on the other. Carry these cards with you, and when you have a spare minute, use them like flash cards (like you may have done when you were learning your multiplication tables). If you do not know how to spell or pronounce a word, you will have a hard time remembering it.
5. Carefully study each diagram and illustration as you progress through the text. Many students ignore these aids, but the author included them to help you understand the material.
6. Summarize what you read. After you finish a paragraph, try to restate the main ideas. Do this again when you finish the chapter. In your mind, identify and review the main concepts of the chapter, then check to see if you are correct. In short, be an active reader. Do not just stare at a page or read it superficially.

Finally, approach each unit of learning with a positive mental attitude. Motivation and perseverance are prime factors in your effort to achieve successful grades. The combined effects of your instructor, the text, the study guide, and your dedicated work will lead to your success in anatomy and physiology.

How to Use the Exercises in This Study Guide

After you have read a chapter and learned all the new vocabulary it contains, begin working with the study guide. Read the overview of the chapter, which summarizes the main points.

Familiarize yourself with the "Topics for Review" section of the overview, which emphasizes the learning objectives that were outlined in the text. Complete the questions and diagrams in the study guide. The questions have been sequenced to follow the chapter outline and headings, and they are divided into small sections to facilitate learning. A variety of questions is offered throughout the study guide to help you cover the material effectively. The following examples are among the exercises that have been included to assist you.

MULTIPLE CHOICE QUESTIONS

Multiple choice questions will offer you many options to select from, but only one answer will be correct. There are two types of multiple choice questions that you may not be familiar with that have been included in this study guide:

1. "None of the above" questions. These questions test your ability to recall rather than recognize the correct answer. You would select the "none of the above" answer only if all of the other possible answers for a particular question were incorrect.
2. Sequence questions. These questions test your ability to arrange a list of structures in the correct order. In this type of question, you are asked to determine the sequence of structures from the various choices given. You will select the structure that would be the third in the specific sequence, as in this example:

   Which one of the following structures would be the third through which food would pass?
   A. Stomach
   B. Mouth
   C. Large intestine
   D. Esophagus
   E. Anus

   The correct answer would be A.

MATCHING QUESTIONS

Matching questions ask you to select the correct answer from a list of options and to write the answer in the space provided.

TRUE OR FALSE QUESTIONS

True or false questions ask you to write "T " in the answer space next to a statement if you feel the statement is correct. If you believe the statement to be incorrect, you will circle the word or words that make the statement incorrect and write the correct word or words in the answer blank.

IDENTIFY THE TERM THAT DOES NOT BELONG

In questions that ask you to identify the term that does not belong, you are given a series of four words. Three words are given that are related to each other in structure or function, and another word is included that has no relationship to or that has an opposing relationship to the other three terms. You are to circle the term that does not relate to the other three terms. An example might be the following:

Iris   Cornea   Stapes   Retina

You would circle "Stapes" because all of the other terms refer to parts of the eye.

FILL-IN-THE-BLANK QUESTIONS

Fill-in-the-blank questions ask you to make judgments about a situation based on the information presented in the chapter. These questions may ask you how you would respond to a situation or what you would suggest as a possible diagnosis when you are given a set of symptoms.

CHARTS

Several charts have been included that correspond to figures in the text. Certain areas of these charts have been omitted so that you can fill them in to test your recall of these important areas.

WORD FINDS

The study guide includes word find puzzles that allow you to identify key terms in the chapter in an interesting and challenging way.

CROSSWORD PUZZLES

Vocabulary words from the "New Words" section at the end of each chapter of the text have been developed into crossword puzzles. This format encourages both recall and proper spelling. Occasionally an exercise will include scrambled words. This, too, encourages recall and spelling.

LABELING EXERCISES

Labeling exercises present diagrams with parts that are not identified. For each of these diagrams, you are to print the name of each numbered part on the corresponding numbered line. You may choose to further distinguish the structures by coloring them with a variety of colors. After you have written down the names of all the structures to be identified, check your answers. When it comes time to review before an examination, you can place a sheet of paper over the answers you have already written on the lines. This procedure will allow you to test yourself a second time without seeing the answers.

After completing the exercises in the study guide, check your answers. If they are not correct, refer to the page listed with the answer and review it for further clarification. If you still do not understand the question or the answer, ask your instructor for further explanation.

If you have difficulty with several questions from one section, refer to the pages given at the end of the section ("If you have had difficulty with this section, review pages..."). After reviewing the section, try to answer the questions again. If you are still having difficulty, talk to your instructor.

How to Use Visual Memory

Visual memory is another important learning tool. If you were asked to picture in your mind an elephant with all of its external parts labeled, you could do that easily. Visual memory is a powerful key to learning. Whenever possible, try to build a memory picture. Remember, a picture is worth a thousand words.

Visual memory works especially well with the sequencing of items such as circulatory pathways and the passageways of air and food. Students who try to learn sequencing by memorizing a list of words do poorly on examinations. If they forget one word in the sequence, then they will forget all the words after the forgotten one as well. However, if you have a strong memory picture, you will be able pick out the important features even if you have forgotten some of the lesser ones.

How to Use Mnemonic Devices

Mnemonic devices are little jingles that you memorize to help you remember things, particularly items in a sequence. If you make up your own, they will stick with you longer. Here are three examples of such devices:
1. "On Old Olympus' towering tops a Finn and German viewed some hops." This mnemonic device is used to remember the order of the cranial nerves; each word begins with the same letter as does the name of one of the nerves.
2. "C. Hopkins CaFe where they serve Mg NaCl." This one reminds you of the chemical symbols for the biologically important electrolytes.
3. "Roy G. Biv." A very popular mnemonic device, this one helps you to remember the order of the colors of the visible light spectrum.

How to Prepare For an Examination

Prepare for an examination far in advance. Actually, your preparation for an examination should begin on the first day of class. Keeping up with your daily assignments makes the final preparation for an examination much easier. You should begin your final preparation at least three nights before a test. Last-minute studying usually means poor results and limited retention of the material. The following suggestions may help you improve your test results:
1. Make sure that you understand and can perform all of the learning objectives for the chapter on which you are being tested.
2. Review the appropriate questions in this study guide. Reviewing is something that you should do after every class and at the end of every study session. It is important to keep going over the material until you have a thorough understanding of the chapter and a rapid recall of its contents. If review becomes a daily habit, studying for the actual examination will not be difficult. Go through each question in the study guide and write down an answer. Do the same for the exercises in which you label each structure on a diagram. If you have already done this as part of your daily review, cover the answers with a piece of paper and quiz yourself again.

3. Check the answers that you have written down against the correct answers in the back of the study guide. Go back and study the areas in the text that refer to questions that you answered incorrectly and then try to answer those questions again. If you still cannot answer a question or label a structure correctly, ask your instructor for help.

4. As you read a chapter, ask yourself what questions you would ask if you were writing a test for that unit. You will most likely ask yourself many of the questions that will show up on your examination.

5. Get a good night's sleep before the test. Staying up late and upsetting your biorhythms will only make you less efficient during the test.

How to Take an Examination

THE DAY OF THE TEST

1. Get up early enough to avoid rushing. Eat appropriately. Your body needs fuel, but a heavy meal just before a test is not a good idea.

2. Keep calm. Briefly look over your notes. If you have properly prepared for the test, there will be no need for last-minute cramming.

3. Make sure that you have everything you need to take the test: pens, pencils, test sheets, and so forth.

4. Allow enough time to get to the examination site. Missing your bus, getting stuck in traffic, or being unable to find a parking space will not put you in a good frame of mind to do well on the examination.

DURING THE EXAMINATION

1. Pay careful attention to the instructions for the test.

2. Note any corrections.

3. Budget your time so that you will be able to finish the test.

4. Ask the instructor for clarification if you do not understand a question or an instruction.

5. Concentrate on your own test paper and do not allow yourself to be distracted by others in the room.

HINTS FOR TAKING A MULTIPLE CHOICE TEST

1. Read each question carefully. Pay attention to each word.

2. Cross out obviously wrong answers and then carefully consider those that are left.

3. Go through the test once and quickly answer the questions you are sure about; then go back over the test and answer the rest of the questions.

4. Fill in the answer spaces completely and make your marks heavy. Erase completely if you make a mistake.

5. If you must guess, stick with your first hunch. Most often students will change right answers to wrong ones.

6. If you will not be penalized for guessing, do not leave any blanks.

HINTS FOR TAKING AN ESSAY TEST

1. Budget time for each question.
2. Write legibly and try to spell words correctly.
3. Be concise, complete, and specific. Do not be repetitious or long-winded.
4. Organize your answer in an outline. This will help you to keep your thoughts organized, and it will also help the person who is grading the test.
5. Answer each questions as thoroughly as you can, but leave some room for possible additions.

HINTS FOR TAKING A LABORATORY PRACTICAL EXAMINATION

Students often have a hard time with this kind of test. Visual memory is very important in this situation. To put it simply, you must be able to identify every structure you have studied. If you are unable to identify a structure, then you will be unable to answer any questions about that structure.

The types of questions that may appear on this sort of examination include the following:
1. Identification of a structure, organ, feature.
2. Description of the function of a structure, organ, feature.
3. Description of the sequence in which air flow, passage of food, elimination of urine, etc. occurs.
4. Disease questions. For example: If the kidney, pancreas, liver, etc. fails, what disease will result?

How to Find Out Why Questions Were Missed on an Examination

AFTER THE EXAMINATION

Go over your test after it has been scored to see what you missed and why you missed it. You can pick up important clues that will help you on future examinations. Ask yourself these questions:
1. Did I miss questions because I did not read them carefully?
2. Did I miss questions because I had gaps in my knowledge?
3. Did I miss questions because I did not understand certain scientific words?
4. Did I miss questions because I did not have a good visual memory of things?

Be sure to go back and learn the things you did not know. Chances are good that these topics will come up on the final examination.

Your grades in other classes will also improve when you apply these study methods. Learning should be fun. With these helpful hints and this study guide, you should be able to achieve the grades you desire in your anatomy and physiology class. Good luck!

Acknowledgments

I wish to express my appreciation to the staff of Mosby, Inc., and especially to June Thompson and Billi Carcheri Sharp for opening this door. My continued admiration and thanks to Gary Thibodeau and Kevin Patton for another outstanding edition of their text. Your time and dedication to science education will hopefully create a better quality of health care in the future.

Special thanks to Randy Fagan for her perseverance and enthusiasm while transposing the written word to typed script.

A. Christine Payne and her computer combined efforts to produce crossword puzzles and word finds for the chapters of this book. Her creativity added the variety necessary to stimulate the learning process.

To my daughter Amanda and my son-in-law Bill, my thanks for your assistance and support throughout this project and my life.

This book is dedicated to the memory of my beloved husband Bill—you will always remain the wind beneath my wings.

Linda Swisher, RN, EdD

Contents

CHAPTER **1**

An Introduction to the Structure and Function of the Body

A command of terminology is necessary for a student to be successful in any area of science. This chapter defines the terms and concepts that are basic to the field of anatomy and physiology. A firm understanding of these ideas will assist you with all future chapters.

The study of anatomy and physiology involves the structure and function of an organism and the relationship of its parts. It begins with a basic organization of the body into different structural levels. Beginning with the smallest level (the cell) and progressing to the largest, most complex level (the system), this chapter familiarizes you with the terminology and the levels of organization necessary to facilitate the study of the body both as parts and as a whole.

It is also important to be able to identify and describe specific body areas or regions as you progress in this field. The anatomical position is used as a reference position when the body is dissected into planes, regions, or cavities. The terms defined in this chapter allow you to describe these areas efficiently and accurately.

Finally, the process of homeostasis is reviewed. This state of relative constancy in the chemical composition of body fluids is necessary for good health. In fact, the very survival of the body depends on the successful maintenance of homeostasis.

TOPICS FOR REVIEW

Before progressing to Chapter 2, you should have an understanding of the structural levels of organization; the planes, regions, and cavities of the body; the terms used to describe these areas, and the concept of homeostasis as it relates to the survival of the species.

STRUCTURAL LEVELS OF ORGANIZATION

Match the term on the left with the proper selection on the right.

_____ 1. Organism
_____ 2. Cells
_____ 3. Tissue
_____ 4. Organ
_____ 5. Systems

A. Many similar cells that act together to perform a common function
B. The most complex units that make up the body
C. A group of several different kinds of tissues arranged to perform a special function
D. Denotes a living thing
E. The smallest living units of structure and function in the body

▶ *If you have had difficulty with this section, review pages 1 and 2.*

ANATOMICAL POSITION

Match the term on the left with the proper selection on the right.

_____ 6. Body
_____ 7. Arms
_____ 8. Feet
_____ 9. Prone
_____ 10. Supine

A. At the sides
B. Face upward
C. Erect
D. Face downward
E. Forward

▶ *If you have had difficulty with this section, review page 2.*

ANATOMICAL DIRECTIONS PLANES OR BODY SECTIONS

Fill in the crossword puzzle.

Across

12. Lower or below
13. Horizontal plane
16. Toward the midline of the body

Down

11. Upper or above
14. Front (abdominal side)
15. Toward the side of the body
17. Farthest from the point of origin of a body point

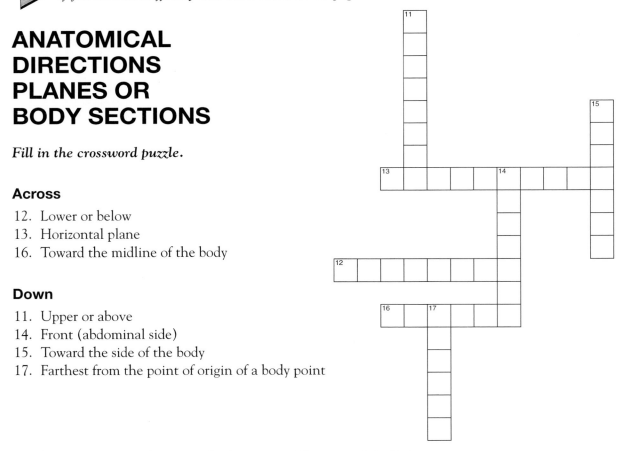

Circle the correct answer.

18. The stomach is (superior or inferior) to the diaphragm.
19. The nose is located on the (anterior or posterior) surface of the body.
20. The lungs lie (medial or lateral) to the heart.
21. The elbow lies (proximal or distal) to the forearm.
22. The skin is (superficial or deep) to the muscles below it.
23. A midsagittal plane divides the body into (equal or unequal) parts.
24. A frontal plane divides the body into (anterior and posterior or superior and inferior) sections.
25. A transverse plane divides the body into (right and left or upper and lower) sections.
26. A coronal plane may also be referred to as a (sagittal or frontal) plane.

 If you have had difficulty with this section, review pages 4-6.

BODY CAVITIES

Select the correct term from the choices given and insert the letter in the answer blank.

A. Ventral cavity   B. Dorsal cavity

_____ 27. Thoracic
_____ 28. Cranial
_____ 29. Abdominal
_____ 30. Pelvic
_____ 31. Mediastinum
_____ 32. Spinal
_____ 33. Pleural

If you have had difficulty with this section, review pages 6-7.

BODY REGIONS

Circle the one that does not belong.

34. Axial	Head	Trunk	Extremities
35. Axillary	Cephalic	Brachial	Antecubital
36. Frontal	Orbital	Plantar	Nasal
37. Carpal	Crural	Plantar	Pedal
38. Cranial	Occipital	Tarsal	Temporal

If you have had difficulty with this section, review pages 8-12.

THE BALANCE OF BODY FUNCTIONS

Fill in the blanks.

39. _____ depends on the body's ability to maintain or restore homeostasis.

Chapter 1: An Introduction to the Structure and Function of the Body   3

40. "Homeostasis" is the term used to describe the relative constancy of the body's _____ _____.

41. The basic type of homeostatic control system in the body is called a _____ _____.

42. Homeostatic control mechanisms are categorized as either _____ or _____ feedback loops.

43. Negative feedback loops tend to _____ conditions.

44. Positive feedback control loops are _____.

45. Changes and functions that occur during the early years are called _____.

46. Changes and functions that occur after young adulthood are called _____.

If you have had difficulty with this section, review pages 12-14.

APPLYING WHAT YOU KNOW

47. Mrs. Fagan has had an appendectomy, and the nurse is preparing to change the dressing. The nurse knows that the appendix is located in the right iliac inguinal region and that the distal portion extends at an angle into the hypogastric region. Place an X on the diagram where the nurse will place the dressing.

48. Mrs. Suchman noticed a lump in her breast. Dr. Reeder noted on Mrs. Suchman's chart that a small mass was located in the left breast, medial to the nipple. Place an X on the diagram where Mrs. Suchman's lump is located.

49. Heather was injured in a bicycle accident. X-ray films revealed that she had a fracture of the right patella. A cast was applied from the distal femoral region to the pedal region. Place an X on the diagram where Heather's cast begins and another where it ends.

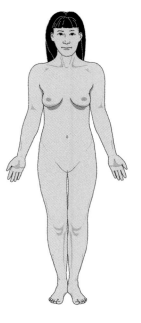

50. WORD FIND

Can you find 18 terms from this chapter? Words may be spelled top to bottom, bottom to top, right to left, left to right, or diagonally.

```
N  H  L  T  E  B  W  N  G  N  M  M  Y  X  A
O  O  H  A  V  U  U  C  L  W  E  P  N  G  L
I  M  U  N  I  T  S  A  I  D  E  M  W  A  L
T  E  R  T  V  C  T  S  I  C  J  S  R  T  K
A  O  N  O  P  T  I  A  I  W  A  T  Y  R  H
Z  S  Q  S  I  R  L  F  A  T  N  R  G  O  W
I  T  W  G  P  R  O  I  R  E  T  S  O  P  F
N  A  A  Z  J  E  E  X  V  E  E  H  L  H  Z
A  S  N  L  M  C  T  P  I  C  P  D  O  Y  T
G  I  C  A  Y  U  O  X  U  M  N  U  I  V  P
R  S  M  R  T  N  U  K  B  S  A  Y  S  V  M
O  R  C  U  R  O  I  R  B  S  Q  L  Y  U  G
L  H  X  E  M  P  M  E  T  S  Y  S  H  V  S
U  W  L  L  Q  D  U  Y  Y  N  E  E  P  J  B
Q  N  Z  P  K  D  B  O  D  C  G  I  N  J  A
```

Anatomy	Organization	Superficial
Atrophy	Physiology	Superior
Homeostasis	Pleural	System
Medial	Posterior	Thoracic
Mediastinum	Proximal	Tissue
Organ	Sagittal	Ventral

DID YOU KNOW?

Many animals produce tears, but only humans weep as a result of emotional stress.

CHECK YOUR KNOWLEDGE

Multiple Choice

Circle the correct answer.

1. The body's continuous ability to respond to changes in the environment and to maintain consistency in the internal environment is called:
    A. Homeostasis
    B. Superficial
    C. Structural levels
    D. None of the above

2. The regions frequently used by health professionals to locate the pain caused by tumors divide the abdomen into four basic areas called:
   A. Planes
   B. Cavities
   C. Pleural
   D. Quadrants
3. Which of the following organs or structures does *not* lie within the mediastinum?
   A. Aorta
   B. Liver
   C. Esophagus
   D. Trachea
4. A lengthwise plane running from front to back that divides the body into right and left sides is called:
   A. Transverse
   B. Coronal
   C. Frontal
   D. Sagittal
5. The study of the functions of living organisms and their parts is called:
   A. Physiology
   B. Chemistry
   C. Biology
   D. None of the above
6. The thoracic portion of the ventral body cavity is separated from the abdominopelvic portion by a muscle called the:
   A. Latissimus dorsi
   B. Rectus femoris
   C. Diaphragm
   D. Pectoralis
7. An organization of varying numbers and kinds of organs arranged together to perform a complex function is called a:
   A. Cell
   B. Tissue
   C. System
   D. Region
8. The plane that divides superior from inferior is known as the ——————————— plane.
   A. Transverse
   B. Sagittal
   C. Frontal
   D. None of the above
9. Which one of the following structures does *not* lie within the abdominal cavity?
   A. Spleen
   B. Most of the small intestine
   C. Urinary bladder
   D. Stomach

10. Which of the following is an example of an upper abdominal region?
    A. Right iliac region
    B. Left hypochondriac region
    C. Left lumbar region
    D. Hypogastric region
11. The dorsal body cavity contains components of the:
    A. Reproductive system
    B. Digestive system
    C. Respiratory system
    D. Nervous system
12. What organ is *not* found in the pelvic cavity?
    A. Bladder
    B. Stomach
    C. Rectum
    D. Colon
13. Similar cells acting together to perform a common function exist at the _____ level of organization.
    A. Organ
    B. Chemical
    C. Tissue
    D. System
14. Which of the following planes would be considered coronal?
    A. A plane that divides the body into anterior and posterior portions
    B. A plane that divides the body into upper and lower portions
    C. A plane that divides the body into right and left portions
    D. A plane that divides the body into superficial and deep portions
15. If your reference point is "nearest the trunk of the body" rather than "farthest from the trunk of the body," where does the elbow lie in relation to the wrist?
    A. Anterior
    B. Posterior
    C. Distal
    D. Proximal
16. In the anatomical position:
    A. The dorsal body cavity is anterior to the ventral
    B. The palms face toward the back of the body
    C. The body is erect
    D. All of the above
17. The buttocks are often used as intramuscular injection sites. This region can be called:
    A. Sacral
    B. Buccal
    C. Cutaneous
    D. Gluteal

18. In the human body, the chest region:
    A. Can be referred to as the thoracic cavity
    B. Is a component of the ventral body cavity
    C. Contains the mediastinum
    D. All of the above
19. Which of the following is *not* a component of the axial subdivision of the body?
    A. Upper extremity
    B. Neck
    C. Trunk
    D. Head
20. A synonym for medial is:
    A. Toward the side
    B. In front of
    C. Midline
    D. Anterior

Matching

Select the most appropriate answer from column B for each item in column A. There is only one correct answer for each item.

Column A

_____ 21. Ventral
_____ 22. Skin
_____ 23. Transverse
_____ 24. Anatomy
_____ 25. Superficial
_____ 26. Pleural
_____ 27. Appendicular
_____ 28. Posterior
_____ 29. Midsagittal
_____ 30. System

Column B

A. Equal
B. Cutaneous
C. Lung
D. Extremities
E. Respiratory
F. Anterior
G. Structure
H. Surface
I. Back
J. Horizontal

Dorsal and Ventral Body Cavities

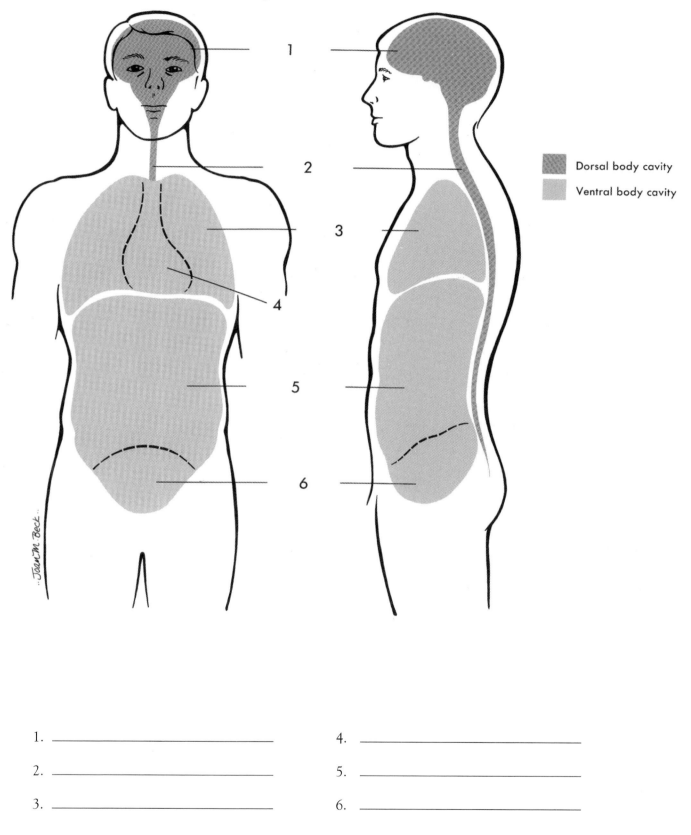

Dorsal body cavity

Ventral body cavity

1. _____   4. _____

2. _____   5. _____

3. _____   6. _____

Directions and Planes of the Body

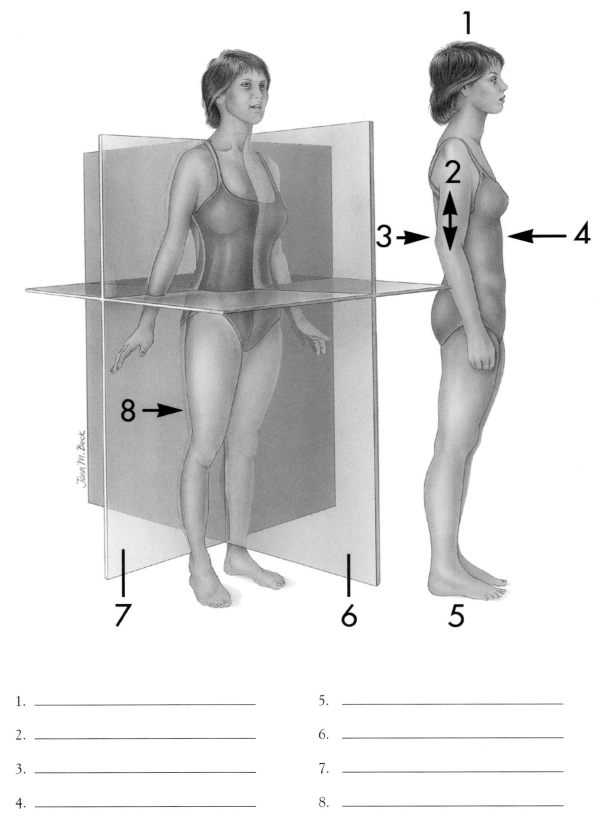

1. _____   5. _____

2. _____   6. _____

3. _____   7. _____

4. _____   8. _____

Regions of the Abdomen

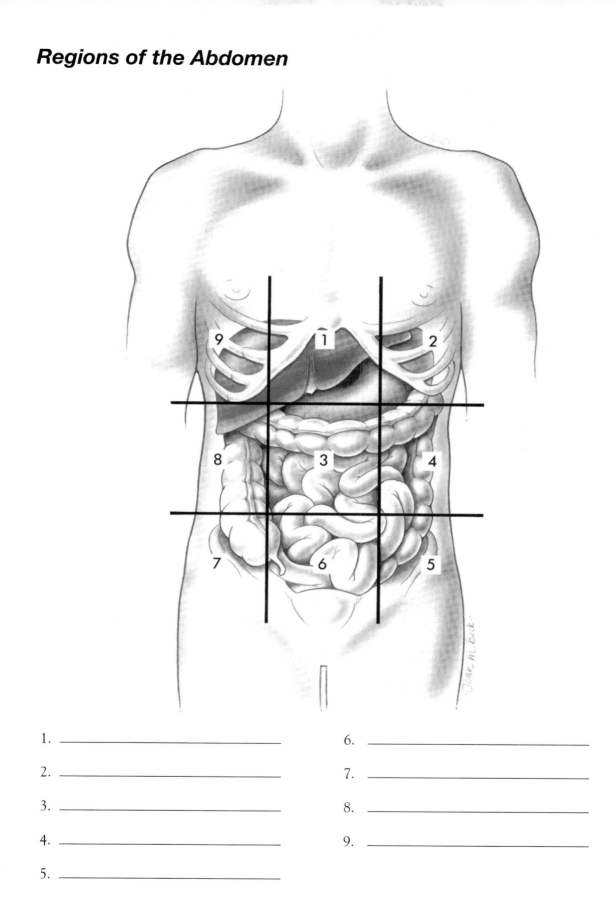

1. _____

2. _____

3. _____

4. _____

5. _____

6. _____

7. _____

8. _____

9. _____

Chapter 1: An Introduction to the Structure and Function of the Body   11

CHAPTER 2

Cells and Tissues

Cells are the smallest structural units of living things. Therefore, because we are living, we are made up of a mass of cells. Human cells, which vary in shape and size, can only be seen under a microscope. The three main parts of a cell are the cytoplasmic membrane, the cytoplasm, and the nucleus. As you review this chapter, you will be amazed at the resemblance of a cell to the body as a whole. You will identify miniature circulatory systems, reproductive systems, digestive systems, power plants (much like muscular systems), and many other structures that will aid in your understanding of these body systems in future chapters.

Cells—just like humans—require water, food, gases, the elimination of wastes, and numerous other substances and processes in order to survive. The movement of these substances into and out of cells is accomplished by two primary methods: passive transport processes and active transport processes. In passive transport processes, no cellular energy is required to effect movement through the cell membrane. However, in active transport processes, cellular energy is required to provide movement through the cell membrane.

The study of cell reproduction completes this chapter's overview of cells. A basic explanation of DNA, "the hereditary molecule," provides a proper respect for the capability of the cell to transmit physical and mental traits from generation to generation. Reproduction of the cell—mitosis—is a complex process made up of several stages. These stages are outlined and diagrammed in the text to facilitate learning.

This chapter concludes with a discussion of tissues that reviews the four main types of tissues: epithelial, connective, muscle, and nervous. Knowledge of the characteristics, location, and function of these tissues is necessary to complete your understanding of the next structural level of organization.

TOPICS FOR REVIEW

Before progressing to Chapter 3, you should have an understanding of the structure and function of the smallest living unit in the body—the cell. Your review should also include the methods by which substances move through the cell membrane and the stages that occur during cell reproduction. As you finish this chapter, you should have an understanding of tonicity and body tissues and the function they perform in the body.

CELLS

Match the term on the left with the proper selection on the right.

Group A

_____ 1. Cytoplasm

_____ 2. Plasma membrane

_____ 3. Cholesterol

_____ 4. Nucleus

_____ 5. Centrioles

A. Component of plasma membrane

B. Controls reproduction of the cell

C. "Living matter"

D. Function in cell reproduction

E. Surrounds and serves as a boundary for cells

Group B

_____ 6. Ribosomes

_____ 7. Endoplasmic reticulum

_____ 8. Mitochondria

_____ 9. Lysosomes

_____ 10. Golgi apparatus

A. "Power plants"

B. "Digestive bags"

C. "Chemical processing and packaging center"

D. "Protein factories"

E. "Smooth and rough"

Fill in the blanks.

11. The numerous small structures that function like organs in a cell are called _____.

12. A procedure performed prior to transplanting an organ from one individual to another is _____ _____.

13. Fine, hairlike extensions found on the exposed or free surfaces of some cells are called _____.

14. The process that uses oxygen to break down glucose and other nutrients to release energy required for cellular work is called _____ or _____ _____.

15. _____ are usually attached to rough endoplasmic reticulum and produce enzymes and other protein compounds.

16. The _____ provide energy-releasing chemical reactions that go on continuously.

17. The organelles that can digest and destroy microbes that invade the cell are called _____.

18. Mucus is an example of a product manufactured by the _____ _____.

19. These rod-shaped structures, _____, play an important role during cell division.

20. _____ _____ are threadlike structures made up of proteins and DNA.

 If you have had difficulty with this section, review pages 22-27.

MOVEMENT OF SUBSTANCES THROUGH CELL MEMBRANES

Circle the correct answer.

21. The energy required for active transport processes is obtained from:
    A. ATP
    B. DNA
    C. Diffusion
    D. Osmosis

22. An example of a passive transport process is:
    A. Permease system
    B. Phagocytosis
    C. Pinocytosis
    D. Diffusion

23. Movement of substances from a region of high concentration to a region of low concentration is known as:
    A. Active transport
    B. Passive transport
    C. Cellular energy
    D. Concentration gradient

24. Osmosis is the _____ of water across a selectively permeable membrane.
    A. Filtration
    B. Equilibrium
    C. Active transport
    D. Diffusion

25. _____ involves the movement of solutes across a selectively permeable membrane by the process of diffusion.
    A. Osmosis
    B. Filtration
    C. Dialysis
    D. Phagocytosis

26. A specialized example of diffusion is:
    A. Osmosis
    B. Permease system
    C. Filtration
    D. All of the above

27. _____ always occurs down a hydrostatic pressure gradient.
    A. Osmosis
    B. Filtration
    C. Dialysis
    D. Facilitated diffusion

28. The uphill movement of a substance through a living cell membrane is:
    A. Osmosis
    B. Diffusion
    C. Active transport process
    D. Passive transport process

29. An example of an active transport process is:
    A. Ion pump
    B. Phagocytosis
    C. Pinocytosis
    D. All of the above
30. An example of a cell that uses phagocytosis is the:
    A. White blood cell
    B. Red blood cell
    C. Muscle cell
    D. Bone cell
31. A saline solution that contains a higher concentration of salt than of living red blood cells would be:
    A. Hypotonic
    B. Hypertonic
    C. Isotonic
    D. Homeostatic
32. A red blood cell becomes engorged with water and will eventually lyse, thereby releasing hemoglobin into the solution. This solution is _____ to the red blood cell.
    A. Hypotonic
    B. Hypertonic
    C. Isotonic
    D. Homeostatic

 If you have had difficulty with this section, review pages 28-32.

CELL REPRODUCTION

*Circle the one that does **not** belong.*

33. DNA	Adenine	Uracil	Thymine
34. Complementary base pairing	Guanine	RNA	Cytosine
35. Anaphase	Specific sequence	Gene	Base pairs
36. RNA	Ribosome	Thymine	Uracil
37. Translation	Protein synthesis	mRNA	Interphase
38. Cleavage furor	Anaphase	Prophase	2 Daughter cells
39. "Resting"	Prophase	Interphase	DNA replication
40. Identical	2 Nuclei	Telophase	Metaphase
41. Metaphase	Prophase	Telophase	Gene

If you have had difficulty with this section, review pages 32-37.

TISSUES

42. Fill in the missing areas of the chart.

TISSUE	LOCATION	FUNCTION
EPITHELIAL		
1. Simple squamous	1A. Alveoli of lungs	1A. _____
	1B. Lining of blood and lymphatic vessels	1B. _____ _____
2. Stratified squamous	2A. _____	2A. Protection
	2B. _____	2B. Protection
3. Simple columnar	3. _____ _____	3. Protection, secretion, absorption
4. _____	4. Urinary bladder	4. Protection
5. Pseudostratified	5. _____	5. Protection
6. Simple cuboidal	6. Glands; kidney tubules	6. _____
CONNECTIVE		
1. Areolar	1. _____	1. Connection
2. _____	2. Under skin	2. Protection, insulation
3. Dense fibrous	3. Tendons; ligaments; fascia; scar tissue	3. _____ _____
4. Bone	4. _____	4. Support, protection
5. Cartilage	5. _____	5. Firm but flexible support
6. Blood	6. Blood vessels	6. _____
7. _____	7. Red bone marrow	7. Blood cell formation
MUSCLE		
1. Skeletal (striated voluntary)	1. _____	1. Movement of bones
2. _____	2. Wall of heart	2. Contraction of heart
3. Smooth	3. _____	3. Movement of substances along ducts; change in diameter of pupils and shape of lens; "gooseflesh"
NERVOUS		
1. _____	1. _____	1. Irritability; conduction

▶ *If you have had difficulty with this section, review Tables 2-6 through 2-8.*

APPLYING WHAT YOU KNOW

43. Mr. Fee's boat capsized, and he was stranded on a deserted shoreline for two days without food or water. When he was found, it was discovered that he had swallowed a great deal of seawater. He was taken to the emergency room in a state of dehydration. In the space below, draw the appearance of Mr. Fee's red blood cells as they would appear to the laboratory technician.

44. A nurse was instructed to dissolve a pill in a small amount of liquid medication. As she dropped the capsule into the liquid, she was interrupted by the telephone. When she returned to the medication cart, she found that the medication had completely dissolved and apparently was scattered evenly throughout the liquid. This phenomenon did not surprise her, since she was aware from her knowledge of cell transport that _____ had created this distribution.

45. Ms. Bence has emphysema. She has been admitted to the hospital and is receiving oxygen per nasal cannula. Emphysema destroys the tiny air sacs in the lungs. These tiny air sacs, called alveoli, provide what function for Ms. Bence?

    _____

    _____

46. Merrily was 5'4" and weighed 115 lbs. She appeared very healthy and fit, yet her doctor advised her that she was "overfat." What might be the explanation for this assessment?

    _____

    _____

    _____

    _____

47. WORD FIND

Can you find 16 terms from this chapter? Words may be spelled top to bottom, bottom to top, right to left, left to right, or diagonally.

```
A   P   D   I   E   V   E   W   N   P   F   E   H   Y   X
I   G   I   Z   N   S   R   L   X   S   T   W   F   Z   S
R   J   V   N   N   T   A   I   L   M   R   P   H   M   F
D   W   U   E   O   O   E   H   B   E   A   D   U   G   F
N   W   I   U   I   C   I   R   P   O   N   N   F   B   W
O   P   U   R   S   H   Y   T   P   O   S   A   W   X   K
H   X   F   O   U   R   Y   T   A   H   L   O   G   A   W
C   L   Z   N   F   O   Y   P   O   R   A   E   M   R   M
O   U   I   X   F   M   L   F   O   S   T   S   T   E   O
T   T   B   Y   I   A   B   C   O   T   I   L   E   S   D
I   V   S   O   D   T   T   M   I   T   O   S   I   S   U
M   N   A   A   I   I   L   E   N   L   N   N   F   R
E   O   K   K   I   D   C   Q   H   B   I   V   I   T   H
E   K   T   X   B   Z   A   E   A   L   S   A   E   C   K
S   B   Z   R   P   M   V   L   X   W   Z   A   Z   C   V
```

Chromatid	Hypotonic	Pinocytosis
Cilia	Interphase	Ribosome
Cuboidal	Mitochondria	Telophase
DNA	Mitosis	Translation
Diffusion	Neuron	
Filtration	Organelle	

DID YOU KNOW?

The largest single cell in the human body is the female sex cell—the ovum. The smallest single cell in the human body is the male sex cell—the sperm.

Cells and Tissues

Fill in the crossword puzzle.

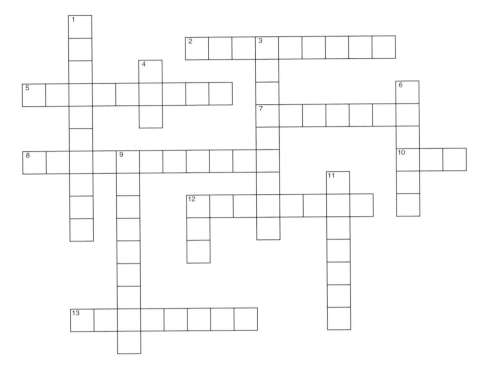

Across

2. Last stage of mitosis
5. Shriveling of cell due to water withdrawal
7. Fat
8. Cartilage cell
10. Ribonucleic acid (abbreviation)
12. Specialized example of diffusion
13. First stage of mitosis

Down

1. Having an osmotic pressure greater than that of the solution of which it is compared
3. Cell organ
4. Energy source for active transport
6. Nerve cell
9. Occurs when substances scatter themselves evenly throughout an available space
11. Reproduction process of most cells
12. Chemical "blueprint" of the body (abbreviation)

CHECK YOUR KNOWLEDGE

Multiple Choice

Circle the correct answer.

1. Which of the following cellular structures has the ability to secrete digestive enzymes?
   A. Lysosomes
   B. Mitochondria
   C. Golgi apparatus
   D. Ribosomes

2. Red blood cells do what when placed in a hypertonic salt solution?
   A. Remain unchanged
   B. Undergo crenation
   C. Lyse
   D. None of the above

3. Which of the following statements is *true* of chromatin granules?
   A. They exist in the cell cytoplasm.
   B. They are made up of DNA.
   C. They form spindle fibers.
   D. All of the above

4. In which stage of mitosis do chromosomes move to opposite ends of the cells along the spindle fibers?
   A. Anaphase
   B. Metaphase
   C. Prophase
   D. Telophase

5. Filtration is a process that involves which of the following?
   A. Active transport
   B. The expenditure of energy
   C. Changes in hydrostatic pressure
   D. All of the above

6. The synthesis of proteins by ribosomes using information encoded in the mRNA molecule is called:
   A. Translation
   B. Transcription
   C. Replication
   D. Crenation

7. Which of the following is *not* an example of connective tissue?
   A. Muscle
   B. Blood
   C. Fat
   D. Bone

8. Which of the following is the most abundant and widely distributed type of body tissue?
   A. Epithelial
   B. Connective
   C. Muscle
   D. Nerve

9. Simple, squamous epithelial tissue is made up of which of the following?
   A. A single layer of long, narrow cells
   B. Several layers of long, narrow cells
   C. A single layer of flat, scale-like cells
   D. Several layers of flat, scale-like cells
10. Which of the following groupings of words correctly describes one of the muscle cell types?
   A. Visceral, striated, involuntary
   B. Skeletal, smooth, voluntary
   C. Cardiac, smooth, involuntary
   D. Skeletal, striated, voluntary

Matching

Select the most appropriate answer from column B for each item in column A. There is only one correct answer for each item.

Column A

_____ 11. Haversian system
_____ 12. Plasma membrane
_____ 13. Neuron
_____ 14. Pinocytosis
_____ 15. Prophase
_____ 16. Adenine
_____ 17. Diffusion
_____ 18. Squamous
_____ 19. Mitochondria
_____ 20. Tendon

Column B

A. Chromatids
B. Thymine
C. Active transport
D. Energy
E. Fibrous
F. Bone
G. Phospholipids
H. Flat
I. Passive transport
J. Axon

Cell Structure

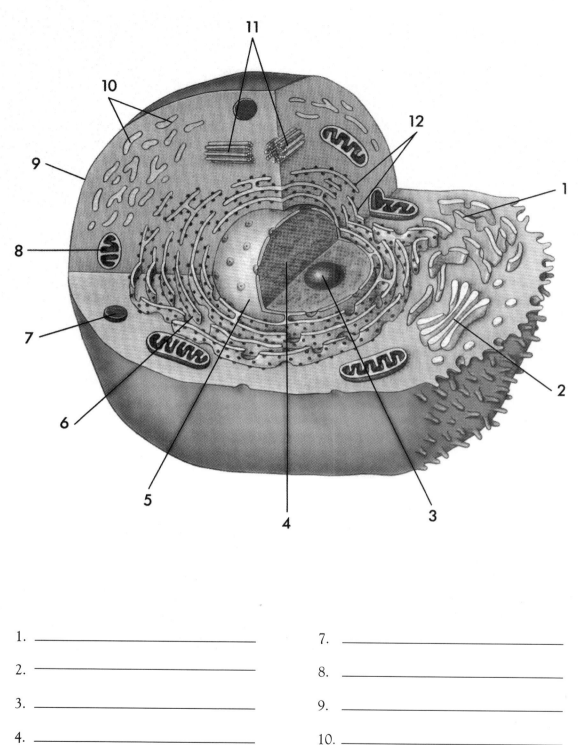

1. _____

2. _____

3. _____

4. _____

5. _____

6. _____

7. _____

8. _____

9. _____

10. _____

11. _____

12. _____

Mitosis

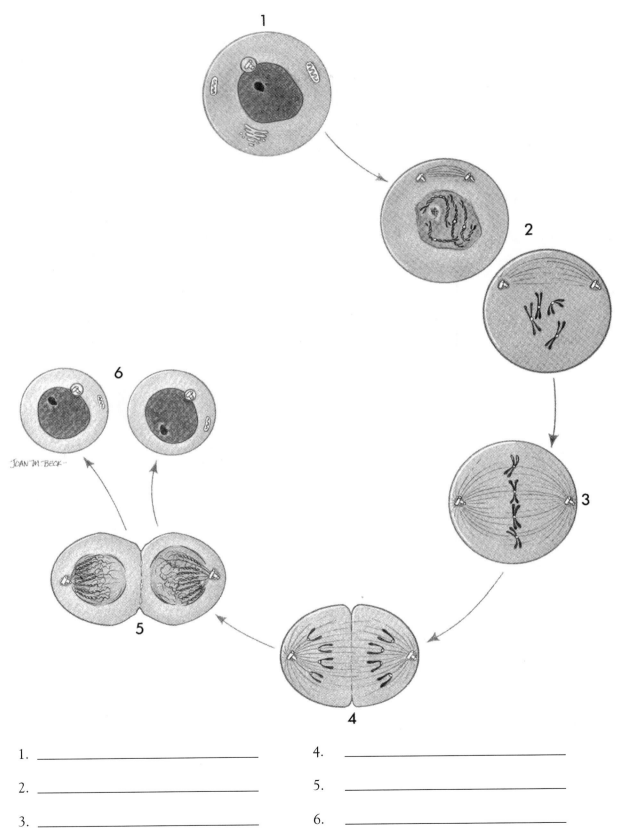

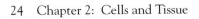

1. _____   4. _____

2. _____   5. _____

3. _____   6. _____

Tissues

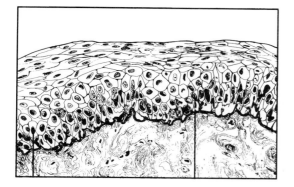

1

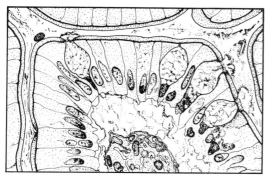

2

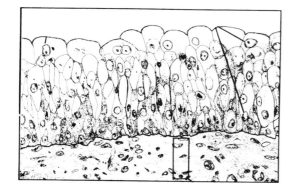

3

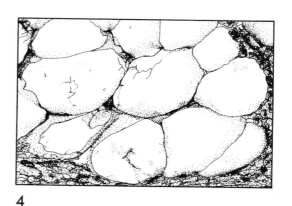

4

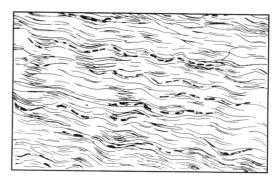

5

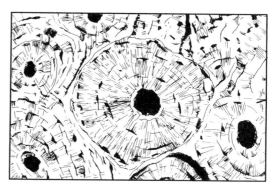

6

1. _____

2. _____

3. _____

4. _____

5. _____

6. _____

Tissues (continued)

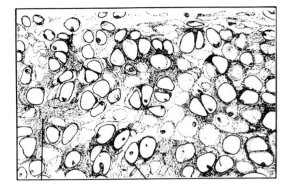

7

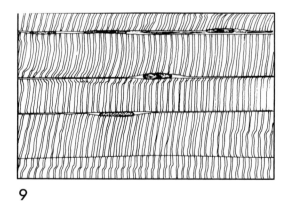

8

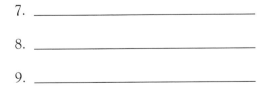

9

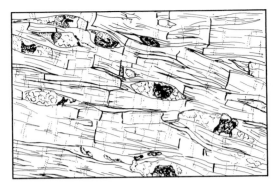

10

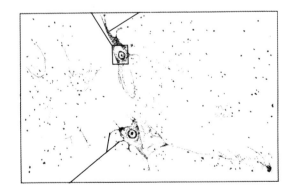

11

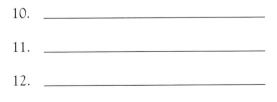

12

7. _____

8. _____

9. _____

10. _____

11. _____

12. _____

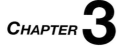

Organ Systems of the Body

A smooth-running automobile is the result of many systems harmoniously working together. The engine, the fuel system, the exhaust system, the brake system, and the cooling system are but a few of the many complex structural units that the automobile as a whole relies on to keep it functioning smoothly. So it is with the human body. We, too, depend on the successful performance of many individual systems working together to create and maintain a healthy human being.

When you have completed your review of the 11 major organ systems and the organs that make up these systems, you will find your understanding of the performance of the body as a whole much more meaningful.

TOPICS FOR REVIEW

Before progressing to Chapter 4, you should have an understanding of the 11 major organ systems and be able to identify the organs that are included in each system.

ORGAN SYSTEMS OF THE BODY

Match the term on the left with the proper selection on the right.

Group A

_____ 1. Integumentary

_____ 2. Skeletal

_____ 3. Muscular

_____ 4. Nervous

_____ 5. Endocrine

A. Hair
B. Spinal cord
C. Hormones
D. Tendons
E. Joints

Group B

_____ 6. Circulatory

_____ 7. Lymphatic

_____ 8. Urinary

_____ 9. Digestive

_____ 10. Respiratory

_____ 11. Reproductive

A. Esophagus
B. Ureters
C. Larynx
D. Genitalia
E. Spleen
F. Capillaries

*Circle the one that does **not** belong.*

12. Pharynx	Trachea	Mouth	Alveoli
13. Uterus	Rectum	Gonads	Prostate
14. Veins	Arteries	Heart	Pancreas
15. Pineal	Bladder	Ureters	Urethra
16. Tendon	Smooth	Joints	Voluntary
17. Pituitary	Brain	Spinal cord	Nerves
18. Cartilage	Joints	Ligaments	Tendons
19. Hormones	Pituitary	Pancreas	Appendix
20. Thymus	Nails	Hair	Oil glands
21. Esophagus	Pharynx	Mouth	Trachea
22. Thymus	Spleen	Tonsils	Liver

Fill in the missing areas of the chart.

SYSTEM	ORGANS	FUNCTIONS
23. Integumentary	23. Skin, nails, hair, sense receptors, sweat glands, oil glands	23. _____ _____ _____
24. Skeletal	24. _____ _____ _____	24. Support, movement, storage of minerals, blood formation
25. Muscular	25. Muscles	25. _____
26. _____	26. Brain, spinal cord, nerves	26. Communication, integration, control, recognition of sensory stimuli
27. Endocrine	27. _____ _____ _____ _____	27. Secretion of hormones; communication, integration, control
28. Circulatory	28. Heart, blood vessels	28. _____
29. Lymphatic	29. _____	29. Transportation, immunity
30. _____	30. Kidneys, ureters, electrolyte bladder, urethra	30. Elimination of wastes, balance, acid-base balance, water balance
31. Digestive	31. _____ _____	31. Digestion of food, absorption of nutrients
32. _____	32. Nose, pharynx, larynx, trachea, bronchi, lungs	32. Exchange of gases in the lungs; regulation of acid-base balance
33. Reproductive	33. _____ _____ _____ _____ _____ _____	33. Survival of species; production of sex cells, fertilization, development, birth; nourishment of offspring; production of hormones

▷ *If you have had difficulty with this section, review pages 58-70.*

UNSCRAMBLE THE WORDS

Unscramble the words.

34. RTAHE

35. IEPLNA

36. EENVR

37. SUHESOPGA

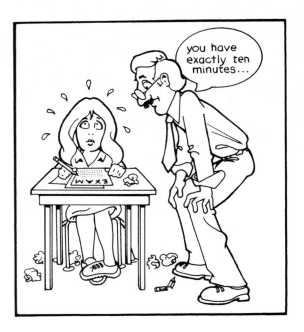

Take the circled letters, unscramble them, and fill in the statement.

The more thoroughly you review this chapter the less

38. ☐☐☐☐☐☐☐ **you will be during your test**

APPLYING WHAT YOU KNOW

39. Myrna was 15 years old and had not yet started menstruating. Her family physician decided to consult two other physicians, each of whom specialized in a different system. Specialists in the areas of _____ and _____ were consulted.

40. Brian was admitted to the hospital with second-degree and third-degree burns that covered 50% of his body. He was placed in isolation, so when Jenny went to visit him, she was required to wear a hospital gown and mask. Why was Brian placed in isolation? Why was Jenny required to wear special attire?

_____

_____

41. WORD FIND

Can you find the 11 organ systems? Words may be spelled top to bottom, bottom to top, right to left, left to right, or diagonally.

```
Y  R  A  T  N  E  M  U  G  E  T  N  I  R  F
H  N  E  R  V  O  U  S  K  I  R  J  M  G  T
L  Y  M  P  H  A  T  I  C  I  S  Y  Y  U  I
B  N  X  Y  R  O  T  A  L  U  C  R  I  C  W
P  E  L  R  E  O  M  J  M  S  O  M  M  P  S
C  C  W  M  A  N  D  L  A  T  E  L  E  K  S
R  R  K  E  M  L  I  U  A  A  V  V  U  K  N
D  K  X  P  D  J  U  R  C  J  I  R  Q  E  M
C  D  B  V  C  V  I  C  C  T  T  K  W  C  X
X  R  Q  Q  D  P  H  C  S  O  I  X  P  A  Z
M  F  M  U  S  Y  D  E  V  U  D  V  Y  K  E
U  E  S  E  C  Z  G  T  Q  D  M  N  E  K  O
P  Y  R  A  N  I  R  U  C  T  C  N  E  W  H
N  H  T  N  D  E  P  S  I  X  A  Q  O  I  E
```

Circulatory	Lymphatic	Respiratory
Digestive	Muscular	Skeletal
Endocrine	Nervous	Urinary
Integumentary	Reproductive	

DID YOU KNOW?

Muscles make up 40% of your body weight. Your skeleton, however, accounts for only 18% of your body weight.

CHECK YOUR KNOWLEDGE

Multiple Choice

Circle the correct answer.

1. Which body system removes waste products from the blood?
   A. Digestive
   B. Endocrine
   C. Circulatory
   D. Urinary

2. Ovaries and testes are considered components of which system?
   A. Reproductive system
   B. Endocrine system
   C. Both A and B
   D. None of the above
3. Which of the following organs is classified as an accessory organ of the digestive system?
   A. Mouth
   B. Esophagus
   C. Tongue
   D. Anal canal
4. Factors in the environment (such as heat, light, pressure, and temperature) that can be recognized by the nervous system are called:
   A. Effectors
   B. Stimuli
   C. Receptors
   D. Nerve impulses
5. Which body system stores the mineral calcium?
   A. Circulatory
   B. Digestive
   C. Lymphatic
   D. Skeletal
6. What is undigested material in the gastrointestinal tract called?
   A. Feces
   B. Urine
   C. Lymph
   D. Blood
7. Which body system produces heat and maintains body posture?
   A. Endocrine
   B. Muscular
   C. Circulatory
   D. Skeletal
8. Which of the following is *not* a function of the integumentary system?
   A. Integration
   B. Temperature regulation
   C. Ability to serve as a sense organ
   D. Protection
9. Which of the following is *not* a component of the digestive system?
   A. Spleen
   B. Liver
   C. Pancreas
   D. Gallbladder

10. When a group of tissues starts working together to perform a common function, what level of organization is achieved?
    A. Systemic
    B. Tissue
    C. Organ
    D. Cellular

Matching

Select the most appropriate answer from column B for each item in column A. There is only one correct answer for each item.

Column A

———— 11. Sweat glands
———— 12. Heart
———— 13. Spleen
———— 14. Vas deferens
———— 15. Bladder
———— 16. Gallbladder
———— 17. Uterine tubes
———— 18. Trachea
———— 19. Spinal cord
———— 20. Adrenals

Column B

A. Endocrine
B. Urinary
C. Integumentary
D. Circulatory
E. Respiratory
F. Digestive
G. Male reproductive
H. Lymphatic
I. Female reproductive
J. Nervous

ORGAN SYSTEMS

Fill in the crossword puzzle.

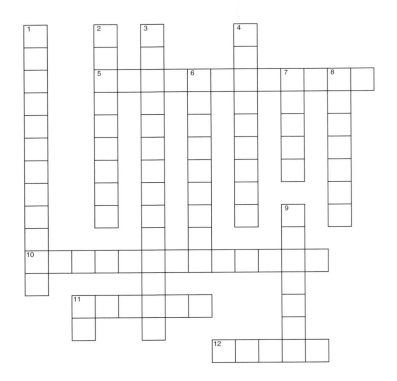

Across

5. Specialized signal of nervous system (two words)
10. Skin
11. Testes and ovaries
12. Undigested residue of digestion

Down

1. Inflammation of the appendix
2. Vulva, penis, and scrotum
3. Heart and blood vessels
4. Subdivision of circulatory system
6. System of hormones
7. Waste product of kidneys
8. Agent that causes change in the activity of a structure
9. Chemical secretion of endocrine system
11. Gastrointestinal tract (abbreviation)

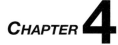

The Integumentary System and Body Membranes

More of our time, attention, and money are spent on this system than on any other one. Every time we look into a mirror, we become aware of the integumentary system as we observe our skin, hair, nails, and the appendages that give luster and comfort to this system. The discussion of the skin begins with the structure and function of the two primary layers—the epidermis and the dermis. It continues with an examination of the appendages of the skin, which include the hair, receptors, nails, sebaceous glands, and sudoriferous glands. Your study of skin concludes with a review of one of the most serious and frequent threats to the skin—burn injury. An understanding of the integumentary system provides you with an appreciation of the danger that severe burns pose to this system.

Membranes are thin sheetlike structures that cover, protect, anchor, and lubricate body surfaces, cavities, and organs. The two major categories of membranes are epithelial and connective. Each type is located in specific areas of the body and is vulnerable to specific disease conditions. Knowledge of the location and function of these membranes prepares you for the study of their relationships to other systems and to the body as a whole.

TOPICS FOR REVIEW

Before progressing to Chapter 5, you should have an understanding of the skin and its appendages. Your review should include the classification of burns and the method used to estimate the percentage of body surface area affected by a burn injury. A knowledge of the types of body membranes, their location, and their function is also necessary as you complete your study of this chapter.

CLASSIFICATION OF BODY MEMBRANES

Select the correct term from the choices given and write the letter in the answer blank.

A. Cutaneous   B. Serous   C. Mucous   D. Synovial

_____ 1. Pleura

_____ 2. Lines joint spaces

_____ 3. Respiratory tract

_____ 4. Skin

_____ 5. Peritoneum

_____ 6. Contains no epithelium

_____ 7. Urinary tract

_____ 8. Lines body surfaces that open directly to the exterior

> *If you have had difficulty with this section, review pages 78-80.*

THE SKIN

Match the term on the left with the proper selection on the right.

Group A

_____ 9. Integumentary system

_____ 10. Epidermis

_____ 11. Dermis

_____ 12. Subcutaneous

_____ 13. Cutaneous membrane

A. Outermost layer of skin
B. Deeper of the two layers of skin
C. Allows for rapid absorption of injected material
D. The skin is the primary organ
E. Composed of dermis and epidermis

Group B

_____ 14. Keratin

_____ 15. Melanin

_____ 16. Stratum corneum

_____ 17. Dermal papillae

_____ 18. Cyanosis

A. Protective protein
B. Blue-gray color of skin resulting from a decrease in oxygen
C. Rows of peg-like projections
D. Brown pigment
E. Outer layer of epidermis

Select the correct term from the choices given and write the letter in the answer blank.

A. Epidermis   B. Dermis

_____ 19. Tightly packed epithelial cells

_____ 20. Nerves

_____ 21. Fingerprints

_____ 22. Blisters

_____ 23. Keratin

36   Chapter 4: The Integumentary System and Body Membranes

_____ 24. Connective tissue
_____ 25. Follicle
_____ 26. Sebaceous gland
_____ 27. Sweat gland
_____ 28. More cellular than other layer

 If you have had difficulty with this section, review pages 80-83.

Fill in the blanks.

29. The three most important functions of the skin are _____,
_____ _____, and _____
_____.

30. _____ prevents the sun's ultraviolet rays from penetrating the interior of the body.

31. The hair of a newborn infant is called _____.

32. Hair growth begins from a small cap-shaped cluster of cells called the _____
_____.

33. The nail body nearest the root has a crescent-shaped white area known as the
_____ or "little moon."

34. The _____ _____ muscle produces "goose pimples."

35. Meissner's corpuscle is generally located rather close to the skin's surface and is capable of detecting sensations of _____ _____.

36. The most numerous, important, and widespread sweat glands in the body are the
_____ sweat glands.

37. The _____ sweat glands are found primarily in the axilla and in the pigmented skin areas around the genitals.

38. _____ has been described as "nature's skin cream."

Circle the correct answer.

39. A first-degree burn (will or will not) blister.
40. A second-degree burn (will or will not) scar.
41. A third-degree burn (will or will not) cause immediate pain.
42. According to the "rule of nines" the body is divided into (9 or 11) areas of 9%.
43. Destruction of the subcutaneous layer occurs in (second- or third-) degree burns.

 If you have had difficulty with this section, review pages 83-90.

UNSCRAMBLE THE WORDS

44. PIDEEMIRS

45. REKTAIN

46. AHIR

47. UGONAL

48. DRTONIDEHYA

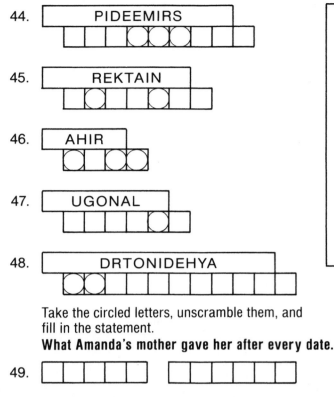

Take the circled letters, unscramble them, and
fill in the statement.
What Amanda's mother gave her after every date.

49.

APPLYING WHAT YOU KNOW

50. Mr. Ziven was admitted to the hospital with second-degree and third-degree burns. Both of the arms, the anterior trunk, the right anterior leg, and the genital region were affected by the burns. The doctor quickly estimated that _____% of Mr. Ziven's body had been burned.

51. Mrs. Tanner complained to her doctor that she had severe pain in her chest and feared that she was having a heart attack. An electrocardiogram revealed nothing unusual, but Mrs. Tanner insisted that every time she took a breath she experienced pain. What might be the cause of Mrs. Tanner's pain?

_____

52. After investigating the scene of a crime, Officer Gorski announced that he had found dermal papillae that would help solve the case. What did he mean?

_____

53. WORD FIND

Can you find 15 terms from this chapter? Words may be spelled top to bottom, bottom to top, right to left, left to right, or diagonally.

```
S  U  D  O  R  I  F  E  R  O  U  S  V  K  R
E  J  U  Q  U  E  S  T  E  C  N  O  H  Y  U
I  S  J  L  M  E  L  A  N  O  C  Y  T  E  H
R  I  M  U  E  N  O  T  I  R  E  P  H  S  B
O  M  K  N  V  A  S  T  R  L  A  N  U  G  O
T  R  G  U  F  G  A  U  C  E  G  O  V  W  D
A  E  A  L  P  R  D  I  O  N  T  F  D  R  N
L  D  V  A  D  M  L  C  P  D  H  S  L  Z  F
I  I  N  Y  N  L  R  L  A  M  E  N  I  R  E
P  P  H  Q  O  N  E  U  X  R  R  F  E  L  G
E  E  Z  F  J  U  M  Y  O  U  U  O  C  C  B
D  Z  P  E  R  J  Y  U  V  F  C  I  I  E  O
G  J  S  I  W  J  S  K  C  D  T  N  O  Z  C
C  O  S  M  Z  M  F  I  B  U  G  U  X  O  J
X  Y  P  M  E  I  W  E  C  V  S  U  G  B  I
```

Apocrine	Epidermis	Mucus
Blister	Follicle	Peritoneum
Cuticle	Lanugo	Pleurisy
Dehydration	Lunula	Serous
Depilatories	Melanocyte	Sudoriferous

DID YOU KNOW?

- Because the dead cells of the epidermis are constantly being worn and washed away, we get a new outer layer of skin every 27 days.
- Your hair will grow 590 miles during your lifetime.
- Your fingernails will grow 84 feet during your lifetime.

CHECK YOUR KNOWLEDGE
Multiple Choice

Circle the correct answer.

1. What is the type of serous membrane that covers organs found in all body cavities called?
   A. Visceral
   B. Pleural
   C. Parietal
   D. Synovial

2. Which of the following statements about synovial membranes is *true*?
   A. They are classified as epithelial.
   B. They line joints.
   C. They contain a parietal layer.
   D. All of the above

3. Which of the following statements about hair follicles is *true*?
   A. Arrector pili muscles are associated with them.
   B. Sudoriferous glands empty into them.
   C. They arise directly from the epidermis layer of the skin.
   D. All of the above

4. Which of the following statements about apocrine glands is *true*?
   A. They can be classified as sudoriferous.
   B. They are found primarily in the armpit and genital regions.
   C. They secrete a thick substance that has a strong odor associated with it.
   D. All of the above

5. Which of the following, if any, is *not* found in the dermis layer of the skin?
   A. Nerves
   B. Melanin
   C. Blood vessels
   D. All of the above are found in the dermis

6. What characterizes second-degree burns?
   A. Blisters
   B. Swelling
   C. Severe pain
   D. All of the above

7. Blackheads can result from the blockage of which of the following glands?
   A. Lacrimal
   B. Sebaceous
   C. Ceruminous
   D. Sudoriferous

8. Keratin is found in which layer of the skin?
   A. Dermis
   B. Epidermis
   C. Subcutaneous
   D. Serous

9. What is the fold of skin that hides the root of a nail called?
   A. Lunula
   B. Body

40   Chapter 4: The Integumentary System and Body Membranes

C. Cuticle

D. Papillae

10. Which of the following is *not* an important function of the skin?

A. Sense organ activity

B. Absorption

C. Protection

D. Temperature regulation

Matching

Select the most appropriate answer from column B for each item in column A. There is only one correct answer for each item.

Column A

_____ 11. Melanin

_____ 12. Epithelial membrane

_____ 13. Pacinian corpuscle

_____ 14. Sebaceous

_____ 15. Waterproofing

_____ 16. Hair

_____ 17. Lunula

_____ 18. Connective tissue membrane

_____ 19. Dermal papillae

_____ 20. Sudoriferous

Column B

A. Fingerprint

B. Pressure

C. Brown pigment

D. Pleura

E. Synovial membrane

F. Perspiration

G. Oil

H. Follicle

I. Keratin

J. Little moon

Completion

Complete the phrases below with the following terms.

A. Skin

B. Eccrine sweat glands

C. Peritonitis

D. Mucous

E. Epidermis

F. Third-degree

G. Pleurisy

H. Sebaceous

I. Hair follicles

J. Receptors

21. The _____ glands secrete oil or sebum for hair and skin.

22. The first line of defense for the body is the _____.

23. The _____ glands work throughout the body, helping to regulate body heat.

24. The _____ burn may involve not only the epidermis and dermis but also muscle tissue.

25. Hair growth requires epidermal, tube-like structures called _____.

26. The outermost and thinnest primary layer of skin is called the _____.

27. A condition that involves the inflammation of the serous membranes that line the chest cavity and cover the lungs is called _____.

28. The _____ membrane lines body surfaces that open directly to the exterior of the body and produces mucus.

29. Specialized nerve endings that make it possible for skin to act as a sense organ are called _____.

30. _____ is a condition in which the serous membranes, which line the abdominal cavity and abdominal organs, are inflamed.

SKIN/BODY MEMBRANES

Fill in the crossword puzzle.

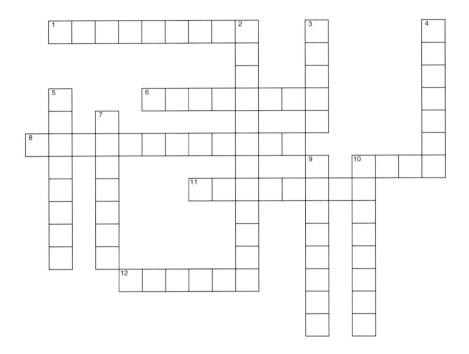

Across

1. Oil gland
6. Bluish gray color of skin due to decreased oxygen
8. "Goose pimples" (two words)
10. Cutaneous
11. Inflammation of the serous membrane that lines the chest and covers the lungs
12. Deeper of the two primary skin layers

Down

2. Sweat gland
3. Cushion-like sac found between moving body parts
4. Brown pigment
5. Forms the lining of serous body cavities
7. Tough waterproof substance that protects body from excess fluid loss
9. Covers the surface of organs found in serous body cavities
10. Membrane that lines joint spaces

Longitudinal Section of the Skin

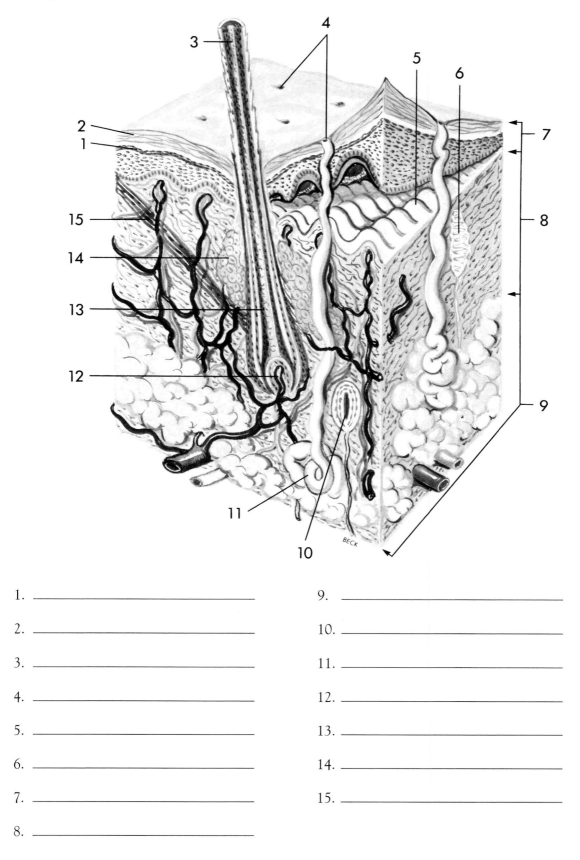

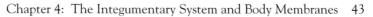

1. _____
2. _____
3. _____
4. _____
5. _____
6. _____
7. _____
8. _____

9. _____
10. _____
11. _____
12. _____
13. _____
14. _____
15. _____

Chapter 4: The Integumentary System and Body Membranes   43

"Rule of Nines" for Estimating Skin Surface Burned

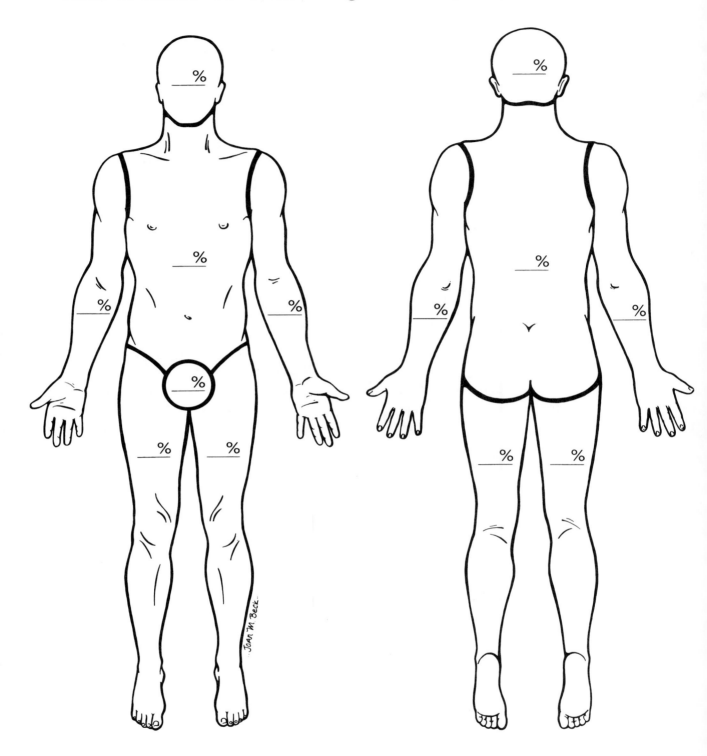

CHAPTER **5**

The Skeletal System

How strange we would look without our skeleton! It is the skeleton that provides us with the rigid, supportive framework that gives shape to our bodies. But this is just the beginning, since it also protects the organs beneath it, maintains the homeostasis of blood calcium, produces blood cells, and assists the muscular system in providing movement for us.

After reviewing the microscopic structures of bone and cartilage, you will understand how skeletal tissues are formed, their differences, and their importance in the human body. Your microscopic investigation will make the study of this system easier as you logically progress from this view to macroscopic bone formation and growth and as you visualize the structure of the long bones.

The skeleton is divided into two main divisions: the axial skeleton and the appendicular skeleton. All of the 206 bones of the human body may be classified into one of these two categories. And, although we can divide the bones neatly by this system, we are still aware that subtle differences exist between men's and women's skeletons. These structural differences provide us with insight into the differences in function between men and women.

Finally, three types of joints exist in the body: synarthroses, amphiarthroses, and diarthroses. It is important to have a knowledge of these joints and to understand how movement is facilitated by these various articulations.

TOPICS FOR REVIEW

Before progressing to Chapter 6, you should familiarize yourself with the functions of the skeletal system, the structure and function of bone and cartilage, bone formation and growth, and the types of joints found in the body. Additionally, your understanding of the skeletal system should enable you to identify the two major subdivisions of the skeleton, the bones found in each area, and any differences that exist between men's and women's skeletons.

FUNCTIONS OF THE SKELETAL SYSTEM
TYPES OF BONES
STRUCTURE OF LONG BONES

Fill in the blanks.

1. There are _____ types of bones.
2. The _____ _____ is the hollow area inside the diaphysis of a bone.
3. The thin layer of cartilage covering each epiphysis is the _____ _____.
4. The _____ lines the medullary cavity of long bones.
5. _____ is the process of blood cell formation.
6. Blood cell formation is a vital process carried on in _____ _____.
7. The _____ is the strong fibrous membrane that covers long bones everywhere except at joint surfaces.
8. Osteoporosis occurs most frequently in _____ _____ _____.
9. Bones serve as a safety-deposit box for _____, a vital substance required for normal nerve and muscle function.
10. As muscles contract and shorten, they pull on bones and thereby _____ them.

▶ *If you have had difficulty with this section, review pages 98 and 103.*

MICROSCOPIC STRUCTURE OF BONE AND CARTILAGE

Match the term on the left with the proper selection on the right.

Group A

_____ 11. Trabeculae
_____ 12. Compact
_____ 13. Spongy
_____ 14. Periosteum
_____ 15. Cartilage

A. Outer covering of bone
B. Dense bone tissue
C. Fibers embedded in a firm gel
D. Needle-like threads of spongy bone
E. Ends of long bones

Group B

_____ 16. Osteocytes
_____ 17. Canaliculi
_____ 18. Lamellae
_____ 19. Chondrocytes
_____ 20. Haversian system

A. Connect lacunae
B. Cartilage cells
C. Structural unit of compact bone
D. Bone cells
E. Ring of bone

▶ *If you have had difficulty with this section, review pages 99-101.*

BONE FORMATION AND GROWTH

If the statement is true, write "T" in the answer blank. If the statement is false, correct the statement by circling the incorrect term and writing the correct term in the answer blank.

_____ 21. When the skeleton forms in a baby before birth, it consists of cartilage and fibrous structures.

_____ 22. Diaphyses are the ends of bones.

_____ 23. Bone-forming cells are known as osteoclasts.

_____ 24. It is the combined action of osteoblasts and osteoclasts that sculpts bones into their adult shapes.

_____ 25. The stresses placed on certain bones during exercise decrease the rate of bone deposition.

_____ 26. The epiphyseal plate can be seen in both external and cutaway views of an adult long bone.

_____ 27. The shaft of a long bone is known as the articulation.

_____ 28. Cartilage in the newborn becomes bone when it is replaced with calcified bone matrix that is deposited by osteoblasts.

_____ 29. When epiphyseal cartilage becomes bone, growth begins.

_____ 30. The epiphyseal cartilage is visible, if present, on x-ray films.

 If you have had difficulty with this section, review pages101-103.

DIVISIONS OF SKELETON

Circle the correct answer.

31. Which one of the following is *not* a part of the axial skeleton?
    A. Scapula
    B. Cranial bones
    C. Vertebra
    D. Ribs
    E. Sternum

32. Which one of the following is *not* a cranial bone?
    A. Frontal
    B. Parietal
    C. Occipital
    D. Lacrimal
    E. Sphenoid

33. Which of the following statements is *not* true?
    A. A baby is born with a straight spine.
    B. In an adult, the sacral and thoracic curves are convex.
    C. The normal curves of the adult spine provide greater strength than does a straight spine.
    D. A curved structure has more strength than a straight one of the same size and materials.

34. True ribs:
    A. Attach to the cartilage of other ribs
    B. Do not attach to the sternum
    C. Attach directly to the sternum without cartilage
    D. Attach directly to the sternum by means of cartilage
35. The bone that runs along the lateral side of your forearm is the:
    A. Humerus
    B. Ulna
    C. Radius
    D. Tibia
36. The shinbone is also known as the:
    A. Fibula
    B. Femur
    C. Tibia
    D. Ulna
37. The bones in the palm of the hand are called:
    A. Metatarsals
    B. Tarsals
    C. Carpals
    D. Metacarpals
38. Which one of the following is *not* a bone of the upper extremity?
    A. Radius
    B. Clavicle
    C. Humerus
    D. Ilium
39. The heel bone is known as the:
    A. Calcaneus
    B. Talus
    C. Metatarsal
    D. Phalanges
40. The mastoid process is part of the _____ bone.
    A. Parietal
    B. Temporal
    C. Occipital
    D. Frontal
41. When a baby learns to walk, the _____ area of the spine becomes concave.
    A. Lumbar
    B. Thoracic
    C. Cervical
    D. Coccyx
42. Which bone is the "funny" bone?
    A. Radius
    B. Ulna
    C. Humerus
    D. Carpal
43. There are _____ pairs of true ribs.
    A. 14
    B. 7

48   Chapter 5: The Skeletal System

C. 5

D. 3

44. The 27 bones in the wrist and the hand allow for more:

   A. Strength

   B. Dexterity

   C. Protection

   D. Red blood cell products

45. The longest bone in the body is the:

   A. Tibia

   B. Fibula

   C. Femur

   D. Humerus

46. Distally, the _____ articulates with the patella.

   A. Femur

   B. Fibula

   C. Tibia

   D. Humerus

47. The _____ bones form the cheek bones.

   A. Mandible

   B. Palatine

   C. Maxillary

   D. Zygomatic

48. In a child, there are five of these bones. In an adult, they are fused into one.

   A. Pelvic bones

   B. Lumbar vertebrae

   C. Sacrum

   D. Carpals

49. The spinal cord enters the cranium through a large hole (foramen magnum) in the _____ bone.

   A. Temporal

   B. Parietal

   C. Occipital

   D. Sphenoid

Circle the one that does not belong.

50. Cervical	Thoracic	Coxal	Coccyx
51. Pelvic girdle	Ankle	Wrist	Axial
52. Frontal	Occipital	Maxilla	Sphenoid
53. Scapula	Pectoral girdle	Ribs	Clavicle
54. Malleus	Vomer	Incus	Stapes
55. Ulna	Ilium	Ischium	Pubis
56. Carpal	Phalanges	Metacarpal	Ethmoid
57. Ethmoid	Parietal	Occipital	Nasal
58. Anvil	Atlas	Axis	Cervical

 If you have had difficulty with this section, review pages 104-115.

DIFFERENCES BETWEEN A MAN'S AND A WOMAN'S SKELETON

Select the correct term from the choices given and write the letter in the answer blank.

A. Male

B. Female

_____ 59. Funnel-shaped pelvis

_____ 60. Broader-shaped pelvis

_____ 61. Osteoporosis occurs more frequently

_____ 62. Larger overall bone structure

_____ 63. Wider pelvic inlet

▶ *If you have had difficulty with this section, review pages 103, 118-119.*

BONE MARKINGS

From the choices given below, match the bone name with the identifying marking. There may be more than one marking for some of the bones.

A. Mastoid
B. Pterygoid process
C. Foramen magnum
D. Sella turcica
E. Mental foramen
F. Conchae
G. Xiphoid process

H. Glenoid cavity
I. Olecranon process
J. Ischium
K. Acetabulum
L. Symphysis pubis
M. Ilium
N. Greater trochanter

O. Medial malleolus
P. Calcaneus
Q. Acromion process
R. Frontal sinuses
S. Condyloid process
T. Tibial tuberosity

_____ 64. Occipital

_____ 65. Sternum

_____ 66. Coxal

_____ 67. Femur

_____ 68. Ulna

_____ 69. Temporal

_____ 70. Tarsals

_____ 71. Sphenoid

_____ 72. Ethmoid

_____ 73. Scapula

_____ 74. Tibia

_____ 75. Frontal

_____ 76. Mandible

▶ *If you have had difficulty with this section, review pages 103-119.*

JOINTS (ARTICULATIONS)

Circle the correct answer.

77. Freely moving joints are (amphiarthroses or diarthroses).

78. The sutures in the skull are (synarthrotic or amphiarthrotic) joints.

79. All (diarthrotic or amphiarthrotic) joints have a joint capsule, a joint cavity, and a layer of cartilage over the ends of the two joining bones.

80. (Ligaments or tendons) grow out of periosteum and attach two bones together.
81. The (articular cartilage or epiphyseal cartilage) absorbs jolts.
82. Gliding joints are the (least movable or most movable) of the diarthrotic joints.
83. The knee is the (largest or smallest) joint.
84. Hinge joints allow motion in (2 or 4) directions.
85. The saddle joint at the base of each of our thumbs allows for greater (strength or mobility).
86. When you rotate your head, you are using a (gliding or pivot) joint.

▶ *If you have had difficulty with this section, review pages 120-126.*

UNSCRAMBLE THE BONES

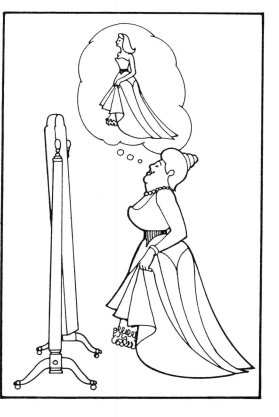

87. E T V E R R B A E

88. B P S U I

89. S C A L U P A

90. I M D B A L N E

91. A P N H G A E L S

Take the circled letters, unscramble them, and fill in the statement.

What the fat lady wore to the ball.

92.

APPLYING WHAT YOU KNOW

93. Mrs. Perine had advanced cancer of the bone. As the disease progressed, Mrs. Perine required several blood transfusions throughout her therapy. One day she asked the doctor to explain the necessity for the transfusions. What explanation might the doctor give to Mrs. Perine?

_____

_____

_____

94. Dr. Kennedy, an orthopedic surgeon, called the admissions office of the hospital to advise that within the next hour he would be admitting a patient with an epiphyseal fracture. Without any other information, the patient is assigned to the pediatric ward. What prompted this assignment?

_____

_____

_____

95. Mrs. Van Skiver, who is 60 years old, noticed when she went in for her physical examination that she was half an inch shorter than she had been on her last visit. Dr. Veazey suggested that Mrs. Van Skiver begin a regimen of dietary supplements of calcium and vitamin D, and he also gave Mrs. Van Skiver a prescription for sex hormone therapy. What bone disease did Dr. Veazey suspect?

_____

96. WORD FIND

Can you find 14 terms from this chapter? Words may be spelled top to bottom, bottom to top, right to left, left to right, or diagonally.

```
A  R  T  I  C  U  L  A  T  I  O  N  N  U  T
M  M  L  T  N  I  N  G  U  I  H  J  N  C  G
P  R  P  E  R  I  O  S  T  E  U  M  A  N  B
H  V  P  G  U  A  T  B  M  E  O  P  R  F  G
I  N  V  R  N  O  B  O  F  S  M  H  X  E  R
A  G  J  O  A  J  P  E  T  O  E  O  H  T  Q
R  U  R  B  X  O  E  E  C  A  S  G  I  S  B
T  S  S  Y  I  M  O  Q  N  U  O  O  L  X  Q
H  J  I  E  A  B  P  U  N  Q  L  E  Q  K  S
R  I  S  I  L  U  C  I  L  A  N  A  C  X  R
O  I  N  A  M  A  S  Q  M  A  Q  K  E  C  T
S  T  S  A  L  C  O  E  T  S  O  U  I  D  G
E  T  S  Y  F  W  L  N  M  P  U  F  N  U  F
S  B  H  Q  H  L  O  U  S  A  R  X  I  T  V
R  P  M  P  A  F  M  G  X  K  D  S  L  G  A
```

Amphiarthroses	Fontanels	Osteoclasts
Articulation	Hemopoiesis	Periosteum
Axial	Lacunae	Sinus
Canaliculi	Lamella	Trabeculae
Compact	Osteoblasts	

DID YOU KNOW?

- The bones of the hands and feet make up more than half of the 206 total bones of the body.
- Approximately 25 million Americans have osteoporosis; four out of five of them are women.
- The bones of the middle ear are mature at birth.

SKELETAL SYSTEM

Fill in the crossword puzzle.

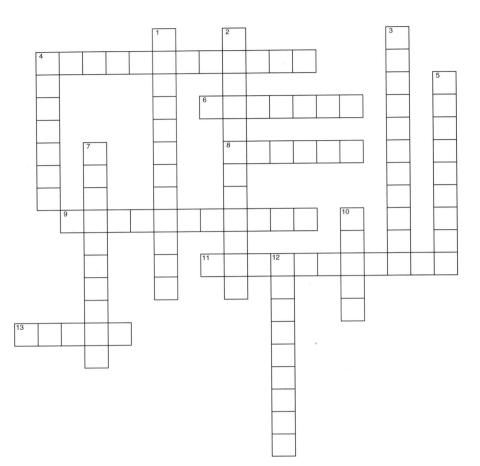

Across

4. Cartilage cells
6. Spaces in bones where osteocytes are found
8. Chest
9. Freely movable joints
11. Process of blood cell formation
13. Space inside cranial bone

Down

1. Joint
2. Suture joints
3. Bone-absorbing cells
4. Type of bone
5. Ends of long bones
7. Covers long bone except at its joint surfaces
10. Division of skeleton
12. Bone cell

CHECK YOUR KNOWLEDGE

Multiple Choice

Circle the correct answer.

1. Which of the following statements about the ribs is *true*?
   A. The first seven pairs attach to the sternum by cartilage.
   B. The last four pairs are called floating ribs because they are free in the front.
   C. The eighth, ninth, and tenth pairs do not move because they are not attached to the sternum.
   D. All of the above statements about the ribs are true.
2. Which of the following is the largest bone in the lower extremities?
   A. Humerus
   B. Ulna
   C. Femur
   D. Radius
3. Yellow bone marrow is made primarily of:
   A. Fatty tissue
   B. Blood cells
   C. Epithelial tissue
   D. Fibrous tissue
4. Which of the following statements regarding the female pelvis is *not* true?
   A. Its shape can be described as broader, shallower, and more basin-like as compared with the pelvis of the male.
   B. Its pelvic inlet (or brim) is usually wider than that of the male pelvis.
   C. Its individual hipbones are usually larger and heavier than those of the male.
   D. All of the above
5. Which of the following statements about the normal curves of the spine (two concave and two convex) are *true*?
   A. They are present at birth.
   B. They extend from the skull to the bottom of the ribcage.
   C. They give the spine strength to support the weight of the rest of the body.
   D. All of the above
6. Which of the following statements about diarthroses is *not* true?
   A. They contain a synovial membrane that secretes a lubricating fluid called synovial fluid.
   B. A diarthrotic joint may permit flexion, extension, abduction, adduction, or rotation.
   C. These joints make up the largest category of body joints.
   D. All of the above
7. Which of the following bones are components of the axial skeletal system?
   A. Ilium, ethmoid, clavicle
   B. Ulna, palatine, occipital
   C. Sacrum, vomer, sphenoid
   D. Scapula, patella, fibula
8. Which of the following bones is *not* classified as a cranial bone?
   A. Sphenoid
   B. Parietal
   C. Palatine
   D. Temporal

9. Which of the following statements characterizes the skeleton of a growing child?
    A. Epiphyses are separated from diaphysis by a layer of cartilage.
    B. Osteoblasts deposit calcium in the gel-like matrix of cartilage.
    C. The periosteum is present.
    D. All of the above
10. What are the joints between the cranial bones called?
    A. Synarthroses
    B. Diarthroses
    C. Amphiarthroses
    D. All of the above

Matching

Select the most appropriate answer from column B for each item in column A. There is only one correct answer for each item.

Column A	Column B
_____ 11. Diarthroses	A. Haversian canal
_____ 12. Spongy bone	B. Trabeculae
_____ 13. Synarthrosis	C. Perpendicular plate
_____ 14. Foramen magnum	D. Red bone marrow
_____ 15. Calcaneus	E. Tarsal
_____ 16. Chondrocyte	F. Ilium
_____ 17. Compact bone	G. Synovial fluid
_____ 18. Ethmoid	H. Cartilage
_____ 19. Coxal	I. Suture
_____ 20. Hemopoiesis	J. Occipital bone

Longitudinal Section of Long Bone

1. _____

2. _____

3. _____

4. _____

5. _____

6. _____

7. _____

8. _____

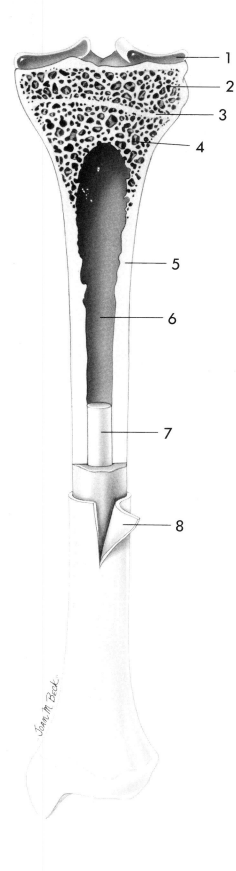

1

2

3

4

5

6

7

8

Anterior View of Skeleton

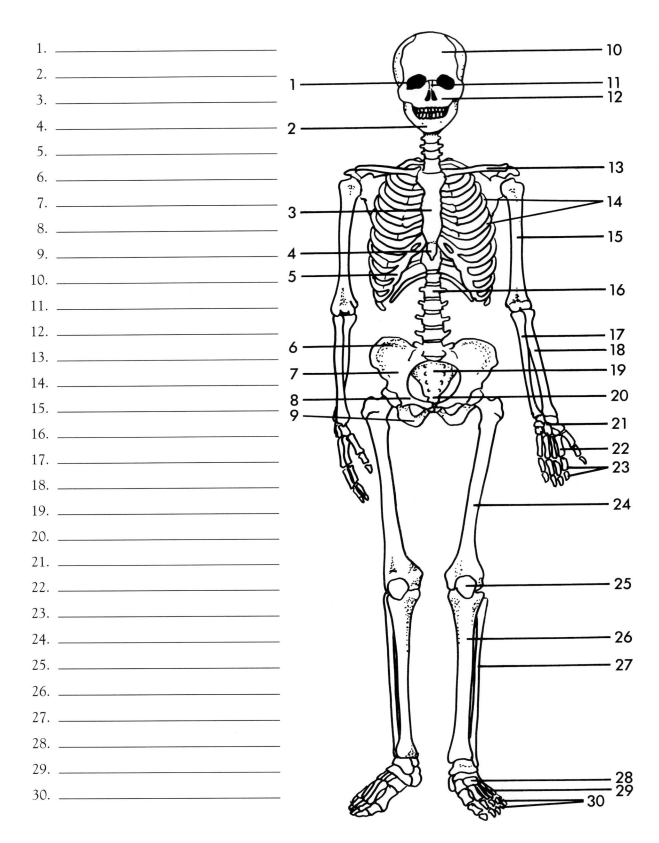

1. _____
2. _____
3. _____
4. _____
5. _____
6. _____
7. _____
8. _____
9. _____
10. _____
11. _____
12. _____
13. _____
14. _____
15. _____
16. _____
17. _____
18. _____
19. _____
20. _____
21. _____
22. _____
23. _____
24. _____
25. _____
26. _____
27. _____
28. _____
29. _____
30. _____

58   Chapter 5: The Skeletal System

Posterior View of Skeleton

1. _____

2. _____

3. _____

4. _____

5. _____

6. _____

7. _____

8. _____

9. _____

10. _____

11. _____

12. _____

13. _____

14. _____

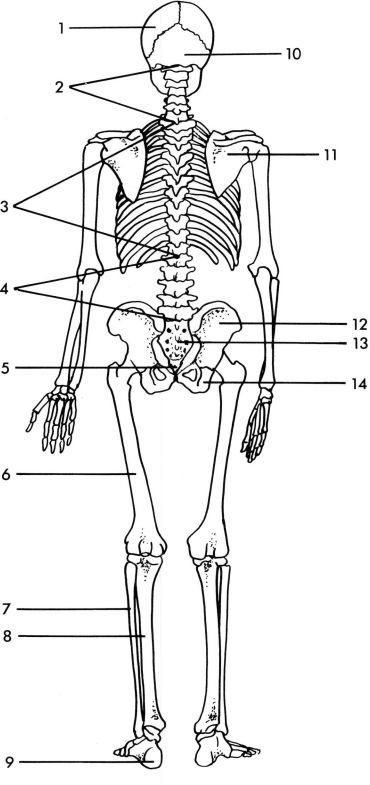

Skull Viewed from the Right Side

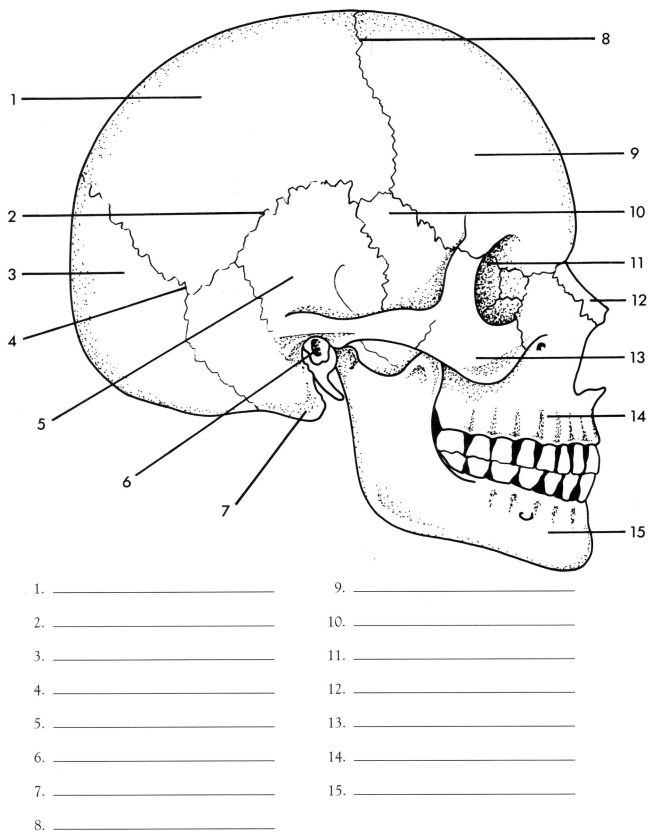

1. _____
2. _____
3. _____
4. _____
5. _____
6. _____
7. _____
8. _____

9. _____
10. _____
11. _____
12. _____
13. _____
14. _____
15. _____

Skull Viewed from the Front

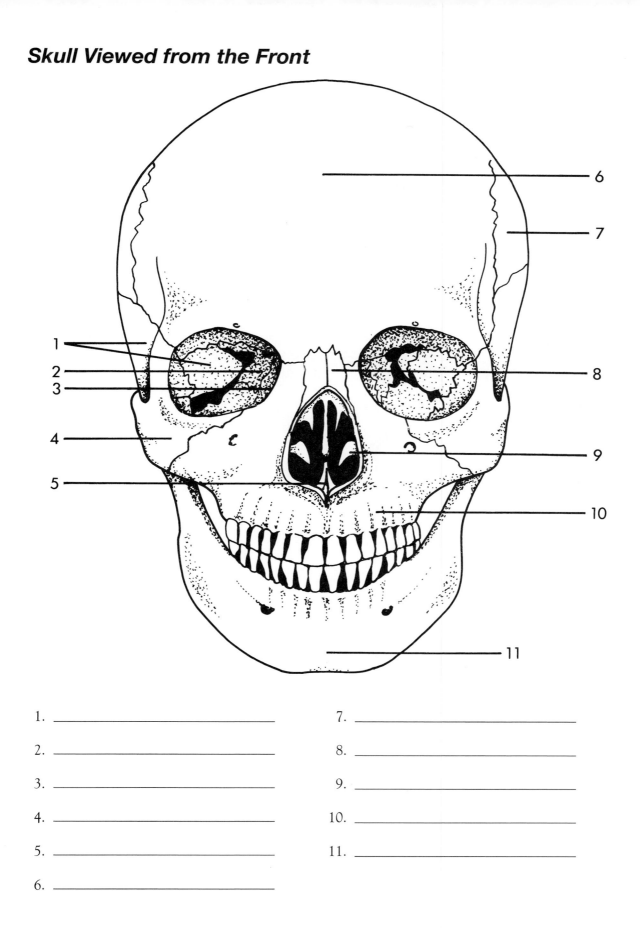

1. _____   7. _____

2. _____   8. _____

3. _____   9. _____

4. _____   10. _____

5. _____   11. _____

6. _____

Structure of a Diarthrotic Joint

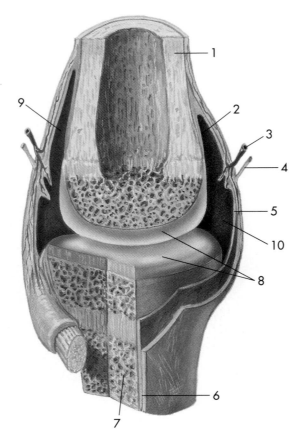

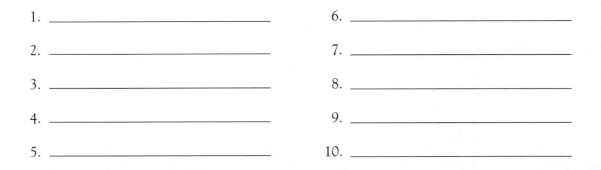

1. _____	6. _____
2. _____	7. _____
3. _____	8. _____
4. _____	9. _____
5. _____	10. _____

CHAPTER 6

The Muscular System

The muscular system is often referred to as the "power system," and rightfully so, because it is this system that provides the motion necessary to move the body and perform organic functions. Just as an automobile relies on the engine to provide motion, the body depends on the muscular system to perform both voluntary and involuntary types of movement. Walking, breathing, and the digestion of food are but a few examples of body functions that require the healthy performance of the muscular system.

Although this system has several functions, its primary purpose is to provide movement or power. Muscles produce power by contracting. The ability of a large muscle or muscle group to contract depends upon the ability of microscopic muscle fibers that contract within the larger muscle. An understanding of these microscopic muscle fibers will assist you as you progress in your study to the larger muscles and muscle groups.

Muscle contractions may be one of several types: isotonic, isometric, twitch, or tetanic. When skeletal or voluntary muscles contract, they provide us with a variety of motions. Flexion, extension, abduction, adduction, and rotation are examples of these movements which provide us with both strength and agility.

Muscles must be used to keep the body healthy and in good condition. Scientific evidence keeps pointing to the fact that the proper use and exercise of muscles may extend longevity. An understanding of the structure and function of the muscular system may, therefore, add quality and quantity to our lives.

TOPICS FOR REVIEW

Before progressing to Chapter 7, you should familiarize yourself with the structure and function of the three major types of muscle tissue. Your review should include the microscopic structure of skeletal muscle tissue, the mechanism by which a muscle is stimulated, the major types of skeletal muscle contractions, and the skeletal muscle groups. Your study should conclude with an understanding of the types of movements produced by skeletal muscle contractions.

MUSCLE TISSUE

Select the correct term from the choices given and write the letter in the answer blank.

A. Skeletal muscle   B. Cardiac muscle   C. Smooth muscle

_____ 1. Striated
_____ 2. Cells branch frequently
_____ 3. Moves food into stomach
_____ 4. Nonstriated
_____ 5. Voluntary
_____ 6. Keeps blood circulating through its vessels
_____ 7. Involuntary
_____ 8. Attaches to bone
_____ 9. Found in hollow internal organs
_____ 10. Maintains normal blood pressure

▶ *If you have had difficulty with this section, review pages 134-135.*

SKELETAL MUSCLES

Match the term on the left with the proper selection on the right.

Group A

_____ 11. Origin
_____ 12. Insertion
_____ 13. Body
_____ 14. Tendons
_____ 15. Bursae

A. The muscle unit, excluding the ends
B. Attachment to the more movable bone
C. Fluid-filled sacs
D. Attachment to more stationary bone
E. Attach muscle to bones

MICROSCOPIC STRUCTURE

Group B

_____ 16. Muscle fibers
_____ 17. Actin
_____ 18. Sarcomere
_____ 19. Myosin
_____ 20. Myofilament

A. Protein that forms thick myofilaments
B. Basic functional unit of skeletal muscle
C. Protein that forms thin myofilaments
D. Microscopic threadlike structures found in skeletal muscle fibers
E. Specialized contractile cells of muscle tissue

▶ *If you have had difficulty with this section, review page 135.*

FUNCTIONS OF SKELETAL MUSCLE

Fill in the blanks.

21. Muscles move bones by _____ on them.
22. As a rule, only the _____ bone moves.
23. The _____ bone moves toward the _____ bone.
24. Of all the muscles contracting simultaneously, the one mainly responsible for producing a particular movement is called the _____ _____ for that movement.
25. As prime movers contract, muscles called _____ relax.
26. The biceps brachii is the prime mover during flexing, and the brachialis is its helper or _____ muscle.
27. We are able to maintain our body position because of a specialized type of skeletal muscle contraction called _____ _____.
28. _____ _____ maintains body posture by counteracting the pull of gravity.
29. A decrease in temperature, a condition known as _____, will drastically affect cellular activity and normal body function.
30. Energy required to produce a muscle contraction is obtained from _____.

 If you have had difficulty with this section, review pages 137-138.

FATIGUE
ROLE OF BODY SYSTEMS
MOTOR UNIT
MUSCLE STIMULUS

If the statement is true, write "T" in the answer blank. If the statement is false, correct the statement by circling the incorrect term and writing the correct term in the answer blank.

_____ 31. The point of contact between the nerve ending and the muscle fiber is called a motor neuron.

_____ 32. A motor neuron together with the cells it innervates is called a motor unit.

_____ 33. If muscle cells are stimulated repeatedly without adequate periods of rest, the strength of the muscle contraction will decrease resulting in fatigue.

_____ 34. The depletion of oxygen in muscle cells during vigorous and prolonged exercise is known as fatigue.

_____ 35. An adequate stimulus will contract a muscle cell completely because of the "must" theory.

_____ 36. When oxygen supplies run low, muscle cells produce ATP and other waste products during contraction.

_____ 37. In a laboratory setting, a single muscle fiber can be isolated and subjected to stimuli of varying intensities so that it can be studied.

_____ 38. The minimal level of stimulation required to cause a fiber to contract is called the threshold stimulus.

_____ 39. Smooth muscles bring about movements by pulling on bones across movable joints.

_____ 40. A nervous system disorder that shuts off impulses to certain skeletal muscles may result in paralysis.

TYPES OF SKELETAL MUSCLE CONTRACTION

Circle the correct answer.

41. When a muscle does not shorten and no movement results, the contraction is:
    A. Isometric
    B. Isotonic
    C. Twitch
    D. Tetanic

42. Walking is an example of which type of contraction?
    A. Isometric
    B. Isotonic
    C. Twitch
    D. Tetanic

43. Pushing against a wall is an example of of which type of contraction?
    A. Isotonic
    B. Isometric
    C. Twitch
    D. Tetanic

44. Endurance training is also known as:
    A. Isometrics
    B. Hypertrophy
    C. Aerobic training
    D. Strength training

45. Benefits of regular exercise include all of the following *except:*
    A. Improved lung function
    B. More efficient heart
    C. Less fatigue
    D. Atrophy

46. Twitch contractions can be easily seen:
    A. In isolated muscles prepared for research
    B. In a great deal of normal muscle activity
    C. During resting periods
    D. None of the above

47. Individual contractions "melt" together to produce a sustained contraction or:
    A. Twitch
    B. Tetanus
    C. Isotonic response
    D. Isometric response

48. In most cases, isotonic contraction of muscle produces movement at a/an:
    A. Insertion
    B. Origin
    C. Joint
    D. Bursa
49. Prolonged inactivity causes muscles to shrink in mass, producing a condition called:
    A. Hypertrophy
    B. Disuse atrophy
    C. Paralysis
    D. Muscle fatigue
50. Muscle hypertrophy can be best enhanced by a program of:
    A. Isotonic exercise
    B. Better posture
    C. High-protein diet
    D. Strength training

 If you have had difficulty with this section, review pages 140-141.

SKELETAL MUSCLE GROUPS

Choose the proper function or functions for the muscles listed below and write the appropriate letter or letters in the answer blank.

A. Flexor	B. Extensor	C. Abductor
D. Adductor	E. Rotator	F. Dorsiflexor or plantar flexor

_____ 51. Deltoid
_____ 52. Tibialis anterior
_____ 53. Gastrocnemius
_____ 54. Biceps brachii
_____ 55. Gluteus medius
_____ 56. Soleus
_____ 57. Iliopsoas
_____ 58. Pectoralis major
_____ 59. Gluteus maximus
_____ 60. Triceps brachii
_____ 61. Sternocleidomastoid
_____ 62. Trapezius
_____ 63. Gracilis

If you have had difficulty with this section, review pages 145-153.

MOVEMENTS PRODUCED BY SKELETAL MUSCLE CONTRACTIONS

Circle the correct answer.

64. A movement that makes the angle between two bones smaller is:
    A. Flexion
    B. Extension
    C. Abduction
    D. Adduction

65. Moving a part toward the midline is:
    A. Flexion
    B. Extension
    C. Abduction
    D. Adduction

66. Moving a part away from the midline is:
    A. Flexion
    B. Extension
    C. Abduction
    D. Adduction

67. When you move your head from side to side as in shaking your head "no," you are
    _____ a muscle group.
    A. Rotating
    B. Pronating
    C. Supinating
    D. Abducting

68. _____ occurs when you turn the palm of your hand from an anterior to a posterior position.
    A. Dorsiflexion
    B. Plantar flexion
    C. Supination
    D. Pronation

69. Dorsiflexion refers to:
    A. Hand movements
    B. Eye movements
    C. Foot movements
    D. Head movements

▶ *If you have had difficulty with this section, review page 150.*

APPLYING WHAT YOU KNOW

70. Casey noticed pain whenever she reached for anything in her cupboards. Her doctor told her that the small fluid-filled sacs in her shoulder were inflamed. What condition did Casey have?

    _____

71. The nurse was preparing an injection for Mrs. Satin. The amount to be given was 2 mL. What area of the body will the nurse most likely select for this injection?

_____

72. Chris was playing football and pulled a band of fibrous connective tissue that attached a muscle to a bone. What is the common term for this tissue?

_____

73. WORD FIND

Can you find 25 muscle terms? Words may be spelled top to bottom, bottom to top, right to left, left to right, or diagonally.

```
G  A  S  T  R  O  C  N  E  M  I  U  S  D  U
M  S  G  I  O  N  O  I  S  N  E  T  X  E  U
U  R  N  N  T  O  M  S  R  B  S  F  D  T  T
S  U  I  S  C  I  B  O  N  T  P  N  E  A  R
C  B  R  E  U  X  V  T  O  O  E  C  L  I  A
L  Q  T  R  D  E  C  O  D  A  C  M  T  R  P
E  T  S  T  B  L  M  N  N  V  I  E  O  T  E
X  F  M  I  A  F  Y  I  E  Y  B  N  I  S  Z
S  I  A  O  V  I  E  C  T  L  S  S  D  I  I
S  Y  H  N  S  S  R  O  T  A  T  O  R  G  U
U  A  M  G  A  R  H  P  A  I  D  J  N  R  S
E  H  A  T  R  O  P  H  Y  L  N  J  T  E  B
L  N  O  H  T  D  E  U  G  I  T  A  F  N  T
O  R  I  G  I  N  O  S  N  V  S  B  Z  Y  L
S  B  V  T  O  J  C  T  R  I  C  E  P  S  S
```

Abductor	Flexion	Soleus
Atrophy	Gastrocnemius	Striated
Biceps	Hamstrings	Synergist
Bursa	Insertion	Tendon
Deltoid	Isometric	Tenosynovitis
Diaphragm	Isotonic	Trapezius
Dorsiflexion	Muscle	Triceps
Extension	Origin	
Fatigue	Rotator	

DID YOU KNOW?

If all of your muscles pulled in one direction, you would have the power to move 25 tons.

THE MUSCULAR SYSTEM

Fill in the crossword puzzle.

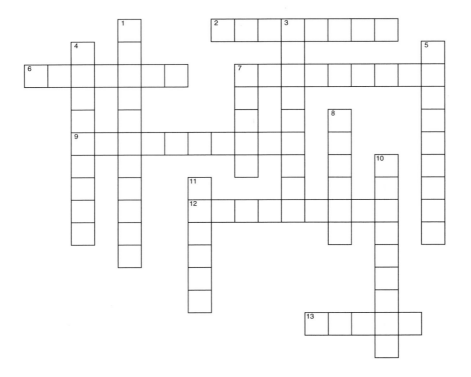

Across

2. Shaking your head "no"
6. Muscle shrinkage
7. Movement toward the body's midline
9. Produces movement opposite to prime movers
12. Movement that makes joint angles larger
13. Small fluid-filled sac between tendons and bones

Down

1. Increase in size
3. Movement away from the body's midline
4. Turning of the palm from an anterior to a posterior position
5. Attachment to the more movable bone
7. Protein that composes myofilaments
8. Attachment to the more stationary bone
10. Assists prime movers with movement
11. Anchors muscles to bones

CHECK YOUR KNOWLEDGE

Multiple Choice

Circle the correct answer.

1. Which of the following statements about a motor unit is *true*?
   A. It consists of a muscle cell group and a motor neuron.
   B. The point of contact between the nerve ending and the muscle fiber is called the neuromuscular junction.
   C. Chemicals generate events within the muscle cell that result in contraction of the muscle cell.
   D. All of the above

2. What is movement of a part away from the midline of the body called?
   A. Abduction
   B. Adduction
   C. Pronation
   D. Plantar flexion

3. According to the sliding filament theory of muscle contraction:
   A. Muscle fibers contain thin myofilaments made of a protein called myosin.
   B. Muscle fibers contain thick myofilaments made up of a protein called actin.
   C. Thin and thick myofilaments move toward each other to cause muscle contraction.
   D. All of the above

4. Which of the following statements about the hamstring group of muscles is *true*?
   A. It includes the rectus femoris.
   B. It flexes the knee and lower leg.
   C. It originates on the pubis.
   D. All of the above

5. What happens if a given muscle cell is stimulated by a threshold stimulus?
   A. It shows an "all or none" response.
   B. It shows a tetanus response.
   C. It shows a subminimal response.
   D. None of the above

6. Which of the following statements about oxygen debt is *true*?
   A. It is caused when excess oxygen is present in the environment.
   B. It causes lactic acid buildup and soreness in muscles.
   C. It can be replaced by slow, shallow breathing.
   D. All of the above

7. What is a quick, jerky response of a given muscle to a single stimulus called?
   A. Isometric
   B. Lockjaw
   C. Tetanus
   D. Twitch

8. Which of the following statements about muscle atrophy is *true*?
   A. It decreases the size of a muscle.
   B. It increases the size of a muscle.
   C. It has no effect on muscle size.
   D. None of the above
9. Which of the following occurs during isometric exercise?
   A. Muscle length remains the same.
   B. Muscle tension remains the same.
   C. Muscle length shortens.
   D. None of the above
10. Which of the following statements about skeletal muscle contraction is *true*?
   A. The attachment to the more stationary bone is called the origin.
   B. The attachment to the more moveable bone is called the insertion.
   C. Both A and B are true
   D. None of the above

True or False

Indicate whether the following statements are true (T) or false (F).

_____ 11. When a part is moved toward the midline, it is called adduction.
_____ 12. An isometric contraction does not shorten or move a muscle.
_____ 13. Dorsiflexion occurs when you turn the palm of your hand from an anterior to a posterior position.
_____ 14. Exercise may cause an increase in muscle size called atrophy.
_____ 15. Isotonic contraction is an example of a contraction used while walking.
_____ 16. If a muscle is overworked without sufficient rest, the result will be fatigue and a decrease in muscle strength.
_____ 17. A bone of insertion moves toward the bone of origin.
_____ 18. A condition in which the body temperature is drastically low is referred to as hyperthermia.
_____ 19. Tetanic contraction is caused by a series of rapid stimuli.
_____ 20. When the angle between two bones becomes smaller, it is called extension.

Muscles Anterior View

1. _____

2. _____

3. _____

4. _____

5. _____

6. _____

7. _____

8. _____

9. _____

10. _____

11. _____

12. _____

13. _____

14. _____

15. _____

16. _____

17. _____

18. _____

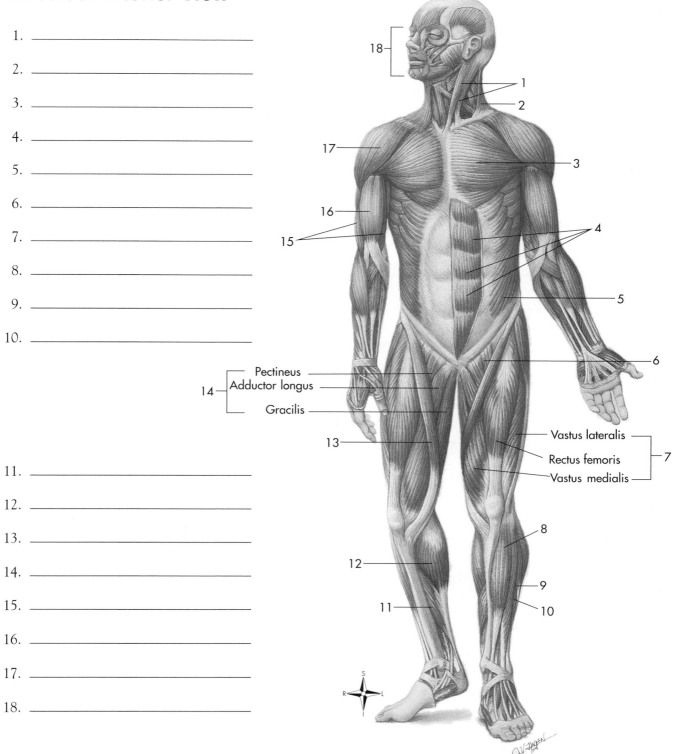

Pectineus

14 — Adductor longus

Gracilis

Vastus lateralis

Rectus femoris   7

Vastus medialis

Muscles Posterior View

1. _____

2. _____

3. _____

4. _____

5. _____

6. _____

7. _____

8. _____

9. _____

10. _____

11. _____

12. _____

13. _____

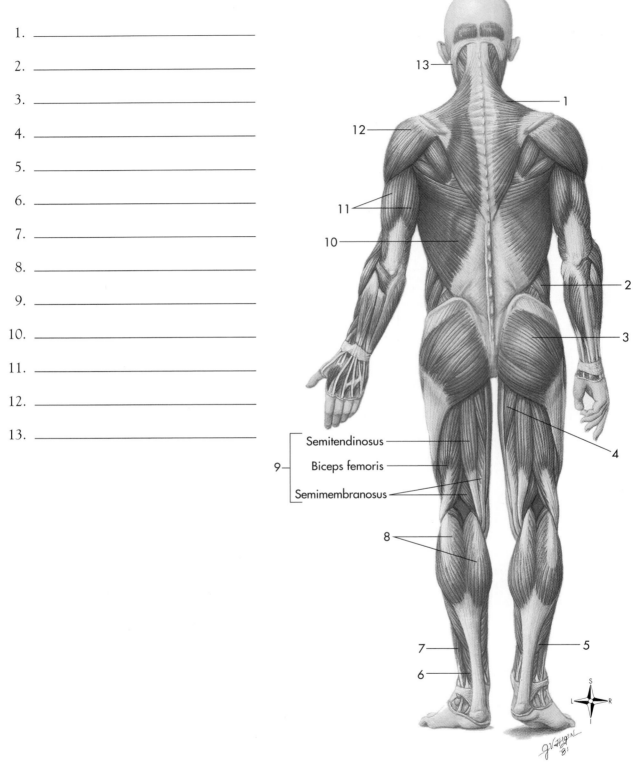

Semitendinosus

9 — Biceps femoris

Semimembranosus

CHAPTER **7**

The Nervous System

The nervous system organizes and coordinates the millions of impulses received each day to make communication with and enjoyment of our environment possible. The functioning unit of the nervous system is the neuron. Three types of neurons—sensory neurons, motor neurons, and interneurons—exist and are classified according to the direction in which they transmit impulses. Nerve impulses travel over routes made up of neurons and provide the rapid communication that is necessary for maintaining life. The central nervous system is made up of the spinal cord and brain. The spinal cord provides access to and from the brain by means of ascending and descending tracts. In addition, the spinal cord functions as the primary reflex center of the body. The brain can be subdivided for easier learning into the brain stem, cerebellum, diencephalon, and cerebrum. These areas provide the extraordinary network necessary to receive, interpret, and respond to the simplest or most complex impulses.

While you concentrate on this chapter, your body is performing a multitude of functions. Fortunately for us, breathing, the beating of the heart, the digestion of food, and most of our other day-to-day processes do not require our supervision or thought. They function automatically, and the division of the nervous system that regulates these functions is known as the autonomic nervous system.

The autonomic nervous system consists of two divisions called the sympathetic system and the parasympathetic system. The sympathetic system functions as an emergency system and prepares us for "fight" or "flight." The parasympathetic system dominates control of many visceral effectors under normal everyday conditions. Together, these two divisions regulate the body's automatic functions in an effort to assist with the maintenance of homeostasis. Your understanding of this chapter will alert you to the complexity and functions of the nervous system and the "automatic pilot" of your body—the autonomic system.

TOPICS FOR REVIEW

Before progressing to Chapter 8, you should review the organs and divisions of the nervous system, the structure and function of the major types of cells in this system, the structure and function of a reflex arc, and the transmission of nerve impulses. Your study should include the anatomy and physiology of the brain and spinal cord and the nerves that extend from these two areas.

Finally, an understanding of the autonomic nervous system and the specific functions of the subdivisions of this system are necessary to complete your review of this chapter.

ORGANS AND DIVISIONS OF THE NERVOUS SYSTEM
CELLS OF THE NERVOUS SYSTEM
NERVES

Match the term on the left with the proper selection on the right.

Group A

_____ 1. Sense organ

_____ 2. Central nervous system

_____ 3. Peripheral nervous system

_____ 4. Autonomic nervous system

A. Subdivision of peripheral nervous system

B. Ear

C. Brain and spinal cord

D. Nerves that extend to the outlying parts of the body

Group B

_____ 5. Dendrite

_____ 6. Schwann cell

_____ 7. Motor neuron

_____ 8. Nodes of Ranvier

_____ 9. Fascicles

_____ 10. Epineurium

A. Indentations between adjacent Schwann cells

B. Branching projection of neuron

C. Also known as "efferent"

D. Forms myelin outside the central nervous system

E. Tough sheath that covers the whole nerve

F. Groups of wrapped axons

CELLS OF NERVOUS SYSTEM

Select the correct term from the choices given and write the letter in the answer blank.

A. Neurons

B. Neuroglia

_____ 11. Axon

_____ 12. Special type of supporting cells

_____ 13. Astrocytes

_____ 14. Sensory

_____ 15. Conduct impulses

_____ 16. Forms the myelin sheath around central nerve fibers

_____ 17. Phagocytosis

_____ 18. Efferent

_____ 19. Multiple sclerosis

_____ 20. Neurilemma

▶ *If you have had difficulty with this section, review pages 164-170.*

REFLEX ARCS

Fill in the blanks.

21. The simplest kind of reflex arc is a _____ _____.
22. Three-neuron arcs consist of all three kinds of neurons: _____,
    _____, and _____.
23. Impulse conduction in a reflex arc normally starts in _____.
24. A _____ is the microscopic space that separates the axon of one neuron from
    the dendrites of another neuron.
25. A _____ is the response to impulse conduction over reflex arcs.
26. Contraction of a muscle that causes it to pull away from an irritating stimulus is known as the
    _____ _____.
27. A _____ is a group of nerve cell bodies located in the peripheral nervous
    system.
28. All _____ lie entirely within the gray matter of the central nervous system.
29. In a patellar reflex, the nerve impulses that reach the quadriceps muscle (the effector) result in
    the classic "_____ _____" response.
30. _____ _____ forms the H-shaped inner core of the spinal
    cord.

 If you have had difficulty with this section, review pages 168-170.

NERVE IMPULSES
THE SYNAPSE

Circle the correct answer.

31. Nerve impulses (do or do not) continually race along every nerve cell's surface.
32. When a stimulus acts on a neuron, it (increases or decreases) the permeability of the stimulated
    point of its membrane to sodium ions.
33. An inward movement of positive ions leaves (a lack or an excess) of negative ions outside.
34. The plasma membrane of the (presynaptic or postsynaptic) neuron makes up a portion of the
    synapse.
35. A synaptic knob is a tiny bulge at the end of the (presynaptic or postsynaptic) neuron's axon.
36. Acetylcholine is an example of a (neurotransmitter or protein molecule receptor).
37. Neurotransmitters are chemicals that allow neurons to (communicate or reproduce) with one
    another.
38. Neurotransmitters are distributed (randomly or specifically) into groups of neurons.
39. Catecholamines may play a role in (sleep or reproduction).
40. Endorphins and enkephalins are neurotransmitters that inhibit the conduction of (fear or pain)
    impulses.

 If you have had difficulty with this section, review pages 171-173.

CENTRAL NERVOUS SYSTEM
DIVISIONS OF THE BRAIN

Circle the correct answer.

41. The portion of the brain stem that joins the spinal cord to the brain is the:
    A. Pons
    B. Cerebellum
    C. Diencephalon
    D. Hypothalamus
    E. Medulla

42. Which one of the following is *not* a function of the brain stem?
    A. Conduction of sensory impulses from the spinal cord to the higher centers of the brain
    B. Conduction of motor impulses from the cerebrum to the spinal cord
    C. Control of heartbeat, respiration, and blood vessel diameter
    D. Containment of centers for speech and memory

43. Which one of the following is *not* part of the diencephalon?
    A. Cerebrum
    B. Thalamus
    C. Hypothalamus
    D. All of the above are correct

44. ADH is produced by the:
    A. Pituitary gland
    B. Medulla
    C. Mammillary bodies
    D. Third ventricle
    E. Hypothalamus

45. Which one of the following is *not* true about the hypothalamus?
    A. It helps control the rate of heartbeat.
    B. It helps control the constriction and dilation of blood vessels.
    C. It helps control the contraction of the stomach and intestines.
    D. It produces releasing hormones that control the release of certain anterior pituitary hormones.
    E. All of the above are true.

46. Which one of the following parts of the brain helps in the association of sensations with emotions and also aids in the arousal or alerting mechanism?
    A. Pons
    B. Hypothalamus
    C. Cerebellum
    D. Thalamus
    E. None of the above

47. Which of the following is *not* true of the cerebrum?
    A. Its lobes correspond to the bones that lie over them.
    B. Its grooves are called gyri.
    C. Most of its gray matter lies on the surface of the cerebrum.
    D. Its outer region is called the cerebral cortex.
    E. Its two hemispheres are connected by a structure called the corpus callosum.

48. Which one of the following is *not* a function of the cerebrum?
   A. Willed movement
   B. Consciousness
   C. Memory
   D. Conscious awareness of sensations
   E. All of the above are functions of the cerebrum
49. The area of the cerebrum responsible for the perception of sound lies in the _____ lobe.
   A. Frontal
   B. Temporal
   C. Occipital
   D. Parietal
50. Visual perception is located in the _____ lobe.
   A. Frontal
   B. Temporal
   C. Parietal
   D. Occipital
   E. None of the above
51. Which one of the following is *not* a function of the cerebellum?
   A. Maintenance of equilibrium
   B. Helps with production of smooth, coordinated movements
   C. Helps maintain normal postures
   D. Associates sensations with emotions
52. Within the interior of the cerebrum are a few islands of gray matter known as:
   A. Fissures
   B. Basal ganglia
   C. Gyri
   D. Myelin
53. A cerebrovascular accident is commonly referred to as (a):
   A. Stroke
   B. Parkinson's disease
   C. Tumor
   D. Multiple sclerosis
54. Parkinson's disease is a disease of the:
   A. Myelin
   B. Axons
   C. Neuroglia
   D. Cerebral nuclei
55. The largest section of the brain is the:
   A. Cerebellum
   B. Pons
   C. Cerebrum
   D. Midbrain

 If you have had difficulty with this section, review pages 174-179.

SPINAL CORD

If the statement is true, write "T" in the answer blank. If the statement is false, correct the statement by circling the incorrect term and writing the correct term in the answer blank.

_____ 56. The spinal cord is approximately 24 to 25 inches long.

_____ 57. The spinal cord ends at the bottom of the sacrum.

_____ 58. The extension of the meninges beyond the cord is convenient for performing CAT scans without danger of injuring the spinal cord.

_____ 59. Bundles of myelinated nerve fibers (dendrites) make up the white outer columns of the spinal cord.

_____ 60. Ascending tracts conduct impulses up the cord to the brain and descending tracts conduct impulses down the cord from the brain.

_____ 61. Tracts are functional organizations in that all the axons that compose a tract serve several functions.

_____ 62. A loss of sensation caused by a spinal cord injury is called paralysis.

▶ *If you have had difficulty with this section, review pages 179-183.*

COVERINGS AND FLUID SPACES OF BRAIN AND SPINAL CORD

Circle the one that does not belong.

63. Meninges	Pia mater	Ventricles	Dura mater
64. Arachnoid	Middle layer	CSF	Cobweb-like
65. CSF	Ventricles	Subarachnoid space	Pia mater
66. Tough	Outer layer	Dura mater	Choroid plexus
67. Brain tumor	Subarachnoid space	CSF	Fourth lumbar vertebra

PERIPHERAL NERVOUS SYSTEM CRANIAL NERVES

68. Fill in the missing areas on the chart below.

NERVE		CONDUCT IMPULSES	FUNCTION
I	_____	From nose to brain	Sense of smell
II	Optic	From eye to brain	_____
III	Oculomotor	_____	Eye movements
IV	_____	From brain to external eye muscles	Eye movements
V	Trigeminal	From skin and mucous membrane of head and from teeth to brain; also from brain to chewing muscles	_____ _____ _____ _____
VI	Abducens	_____	Eye movements
VII	Facial	From taste buds of tongue to brain; from brain to face muscles	_____ _____
VIII	_____	From ear to brain	Hearing; sense of balance
IX	Glossopharyngeal	_____ _____ _____	Sensations of throat, taste, swallowing movements, secretion of saliva
X	_____	From throat, larynx, and organs in thoracic and abdominal cavities to brain; also from brain to muscles of throat and to organs in thoracic and abdominal cavities	Sensations of throat, larynx, and of thoracic and abdominal organs; swallowing, voice production, slowing of heartbeat, acceleration of peristalsis (gut movements)
XI	Accessory	From brain to certain shoulder and neck muscles	_____ _____
XII	_____	From brain to muscles of tongue	Tongue movements

▶ *If you have had difficulty with this section, review page 188, Table 7-2.*

CRANIAL NERVES
SPINAL NERVES

Select the correct term from the choices given and write its letter in the answer blank.

    A. Cranial nerves   B. Spinal nerves

_____ 69. 12 pair

_____ 70. Dermatome

_____ 71. Vagus

_____ 72. Shingles

_____ 73. 31 pair

_____ 74. Optic

_____ 75. C1

_____ 76. Plexus

▷ *If you have had difficulty with this section, review pages 186-195.*

AUTONOMIC NERVOUS SYSTEM

Match the term on the left with the proper selection on the right.

_____ 77. Autonomic nervous system

_____ 78. Autonomic neurons

_____ 79. Preganglionic neurons

_____ 80. Visceral effectors

_____ 81. Sympathetic system

_____ 82. Somatic nervous system

A. Division of ANS

B. Tissues to which autonomic neurons conduct impulses

C. Voluntary actions

D. Regulates body's involuntary functions

E. Motor neurons that make up the ANS

F. Conduct impulses between the spinal cord and a ganglion

SYMPATHETIC NERVOUS SYSTEM
PARASYMPATHETIC NERVOUS SYSTEM

Circle the correct answer.

83. Dendrites and cell bodies of sympathetic preganglionic neurons are located in the:

    A. Brain stem and sacral portion of the spinal cord

    B. Sympathetic ganglia

    C. Gray matter of the thoracic and upper lumbar segments of the spinal cord

    D. Ganglia close to effectors

84. Which of the following statements is *not* correct?

    A. Sympathetic preganglionic neurons have their cell bodies located in the lateral gray column of certain parts of the spinal cord.

    B. Sympathetic preganglionic axons pass along the dorsal root of certain spinal nerves.

    C. There are synapses within sympathetic ganglia.

    D. Sympathetic responses are usually widespread, involving many organs.

85. Another name for the parasympathetic nervous system is:
    A. Thoracolumbar
    B. Craniosacral
    C. Visceral
    D. ANS
    E. Cholinergic
86. Which of the following statements is *not* correct?
    A. Sympathetic postganglionic neurons have their dendrites and cell bodies in sympathetic ganglia or collateral ganglia.
    B. Sympathetic ganglions are located in front of and at each side of the spinal column.
    C. Separate autonomic nerves distribute many sympathetic postganglionic axons to various internal organs.
    D. Very few sympathetic preganglionic axons synapse with postganglionic neurons.
87. Sympathetic stimulation usually results in:
    A. Response by numerous organs
    B. Response by only one organ
    C. Increased peristalsis
    D. Constriction of pupils
88. Parasympathetic stimulation frequently results in:
    A. Response by only one organ
    B. Responses by numerous organs
    C. The fight or flight syndrome
    D. Increased heartbeat

Select the correct term from the choices given and write the letter in the answer blank.

A. Sympathetic control   B. Parasympathetic control

_____ 89. Constricts pupils
_____ 90. Produces "goose pimples"
_____ 91. Increases sweat secretion
_____ 92. Increases secretion of digestive juices
_____ 93. Constricts blood vessels
_____ 94. Slows heartbeat
_____ 95. Relaxes bladder
_____ 96. Increases epinephrine secretion
_____ 97. Increases peristalsis
_____ 98. Stimulates lens for near vision

If you have had difficulty with this section, review pages 188-193.

AUTONOMIC NEUROTRANSMITTERS
AUTONOMIC NERVOUS SYSTEM AS A WHOLE

Fill in the blanks.

99. Sympathetic preganglionic axons release the neurotransmitter _____.

100. Axons that release norepinephrine are classified as _____
_____.

101. Axons that release acetylcholine are classified as _____ _____.

102. The function of the autonomic nervous system is to regulate the body's involuntary functions in ways that maintain or restore _____.

103. Your _____ _____ is determined by the combined forces of the sympathetic and parasympathetic nervous system.

104. According to some physiologists, meditation leads to _____ sympathetic activity and changes opposite to those of the "fight or flight" syndrome.

▶ *If you have had difficulty with this section, review page 194.*

UNSCRAMBLE THE WORDS

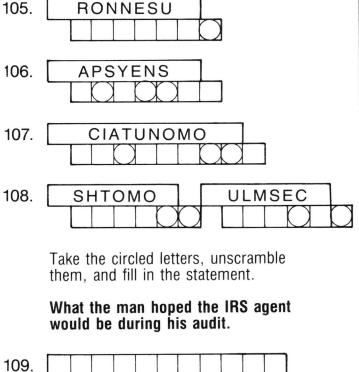

105. RONNESU

106. APSYENS

107. CIATUNOMO

108. SHTOMO   ULMSEC

Take the circled letters, unscramble them, and fill in the statement.

What the man hoped the IRS agent would be during his audit.

109. ☐☐☐☐☐☐☐☐☐☐☐☐☐

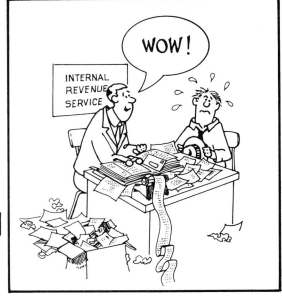

WOW!

INTERNAL REVENUE SERVICE

84   Chapter 7: The Nervous System

APPLYING WHAT YOU KNOW

110. Mr. Wolf suffered a cerebrovascular accident and it was determined that the damage affected the left side of his cerebrum. On which side of his body will he most likely notice any paralysis?

_____

111. Baby Dania was born with an excessive accumulation of cerebrospinal fluid in the ventricles. A catheter was placed in the ventricle and the fluid was drained by means of a shunt into the circulatory bloodstream. What condition does this medical history describe?

_____

112. Mrs. Muhlenkamp looked out her window to see a man trapped under the wheel of a car. Although slightly built, Mrs. Muhlenkamp rushed to the car, lifted it, and saved the man underneath the wheel. What division of the autonomic nervous system made this seemingly impossible task possible?

_____

113. Madison's heart raced and her palms became clammy as she watched the monster movie at the local theater. When the movie was over, however, she told her friends that she was not afraid at all. She appeared to be as calm as before the movie. What division of the autonomic nervous system made this possible?

_____

114. Bill is going to his boss for his annual evaluation. He is planning to ask for a raise and hopes the evaluation will be good. Which subdivision of the autonomic nervous system will be active during this conference? Should he have a large meal before his appointment? Support your answer with facts from the chapter.

_____

115. WORD FIND

Can you find 14 terms from this chapter? Words may be spelled top to bottom, bottom to top, right to left, left to right, or diagonally.

```
M C C D Q S Y N A P S E Q G O
E N A Q D W H N W E J N A L W
S R O T P E C E R Y Z N I S M
I D S X E K N O K X G G C Y Y
J O T R A C T D F L O N E N A
R P W E K O H X I D A L H A M
F A L O N A Y O E I I I X P C
C M Z I F D N N L N G Z U T Z
S I N V C G D G Z A N A K I P
G N A T Z R O W V A M Y T C O
K E N D O R P H I N S I L C X
C P Q G C J X F J D Q S N L F
X U L I H I G Q A N S W O E U
A I M H Q E X K D B W Y T F S
A A D A X O C K G B F H B T K
```

Axon	Glia	Serotonin
Catecholamines	Microglia	Synapse
Dopamine	Myelin	Synaptic cleft
Endorphins	Oligodendroglia	Tract
Ganglion	Receptors	

DID YOU KNOW?

Although all pain is felt and interpreted in the brain, it has no pain sensation itself—even when cut!

THE NERVOUS SYSTEM

Fill in the crossword puzzle.

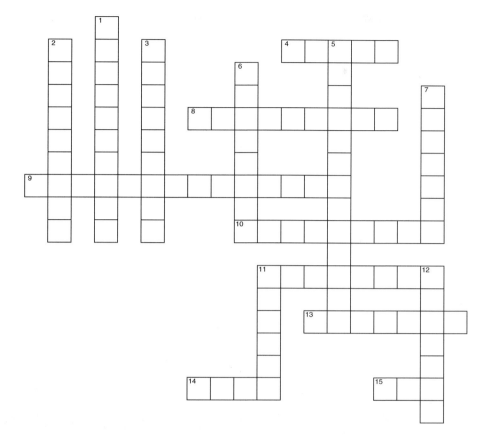

Across

4. Bundle of axons located within the central nervous system
8. Transmits impulses toward the cell body
9. Neurons that conduct impulses from a ganglion
10. Astrocytes
11. Pia mater
13. Nerve cells
14. Transmits impulses away from the cell body
15. Peripheral nervous system (abbreviation)

Down

1. Neuroglia
2. Peripheral beginning of a sensory neuron's dendrite
3. Two-neuron arc (two words)
5. Neurotransmitter
6. Cluster of nerve cell bodies outside the central nervous system
7. Area of brain stem
11. Fatty substance found around some nerve fibers
12. Where impulses are transmitted from one neuron to another

CHECK YOUR KNOWLEDGE

Multiple Choice

Circle the correct answer.

1. What are neurons that pick up sensations from receptors and carry them into the brain or spinal cord called?
   A. Motor neurons
   B. Central neurons
   C. Interneurons
   D. Sensory neurons
2. What are brain cavities that are filled with cerebrospinal fluid called?
   A. Hydrocephalics
   B. Ventricles
   C. Mater
   D. Meninges
3. What is the innermost layer of connective tissue that surrounds the brain and spinal cord?
   A. Pia mater
   B. Dura mater
   C. Arachnoid mater
   D. Pons mater
4. A nurse is caring for a patient with a tumor of the cerebellum. In view of the functions of this part of the brain, which of the following symptoms should the nurse expect to observe?
   A. Irregular heartbeat and increased blood pressure
   B. Inability to coordinate body movements
   C. Loss of speech
   D. Inability to control emotions
5. What occurs as a result of stimulation of the sympathetic nervous system?
   A. Accelerated heart rate
   B. Constriction of blood vessels in skeletal muscles
   C. Increased peristalsis
   D. All of the above
6. The autonomic neurotransmitter called acetylcholine is released by the:
   A. Sympathetic preganglionic axon
   B. Parasympathetic preganglionic axon
   C. Parasympathetic postganglionic axon
   D. All of the above
7. Which of the following statements about Schwann cells is *true*?
   A. They are found in the PNS.
   B. They produce myelin.
   C. They are separated by nodes of Ranvier.
   D. All of the above
8. What are areas of the neuron that secrete neurotransmitters called?
   A. Synapses
   B. Synaptic clefts
   C. Synaptic knobs
   D. Gliomas

9. Which of the following statements about the neural tissues called tracts is *true*?
   A. They are located outside of the central nervous system.
   B. They appear gray.
   C. When carrying messages upward they are called ascending, and when carrying messages downward they are called descending.
   D. All of the above

10. Which of the following statements about the autonomic division of the nervous system is *true*?
   A. It is composed of two divisions: the sympathetic and parasympathetic.
   B. Autonomic neurotransmitters assist the system in its effort to elicit responses.
   C. The system regulates the body's involuntary functions.
   D. All of the above

Matching

Select the most appropriate answer from column B for each item in column A. There is only one correct answer for each item.

Column A	Column B
_____ 11. Tract	A. Transmits away from cell body
_____ 12. Axon	B. Interneuron
_____ 13. Brain stem	C. White matter
_____ 14. Neurotransmitter	D. Cranial nerve
_____ 15. Reflex arc	E. Thalamus
_____ 16. Skin map	F. Glioma
_____ 17. Brain tumor	G. Parkinson's disease
_____ 18. Diencephalon	H. Acetylcholine
_____ 19. Vagus	I. Dermatome
_____ 20. Dopamine	J. Medulla oblongata

Neuron

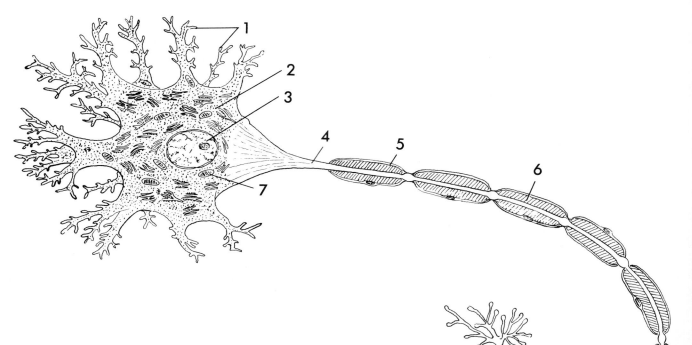

1. _____   5. _____

2. _____   6. _____

3. _____   7. _____

4. _____

Cranial Nerves

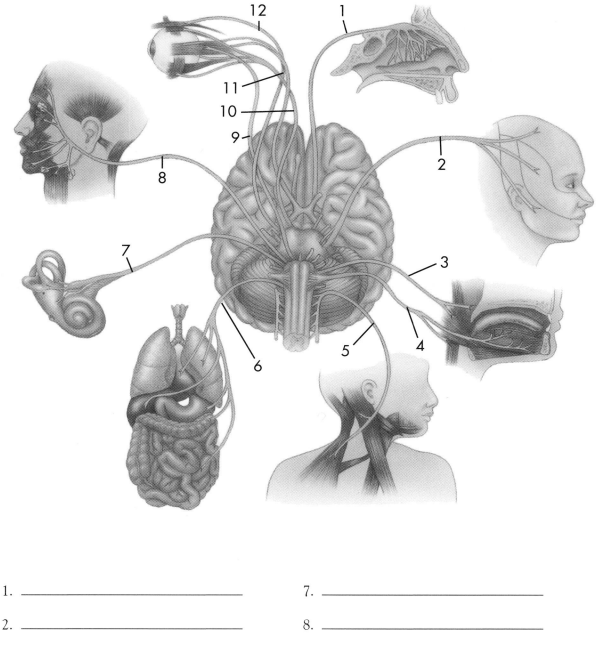

1. _____

2. _____

3. _____

4. _____

5. _____

6. _____

7. _____

8. _____

9. _____

10. _____

11. _____

12. _____

Neural Pathway Involved in the Patellar Reflex

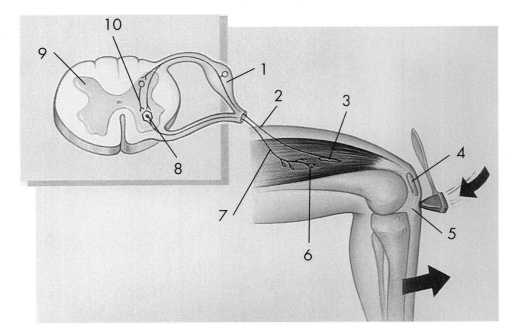

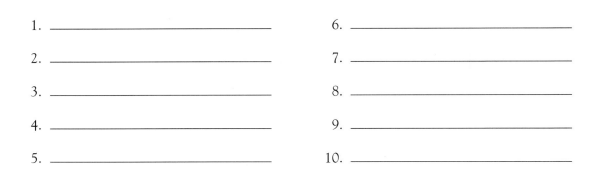

1. _____		6. _____
2. _____		7. _____
3. _____		8. _____
4. _____		9. _____
5. _____		10. _____

The Cerebrum

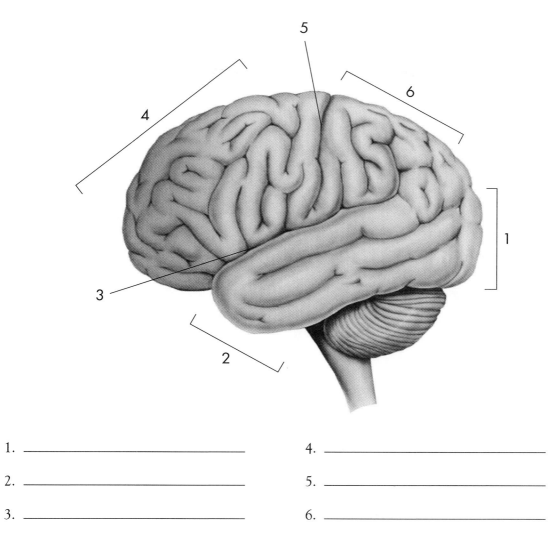

1. _____

2. _____

3. _____

4. _____

5. _____

6. _____

Sagittal Section of the Central Nervous System

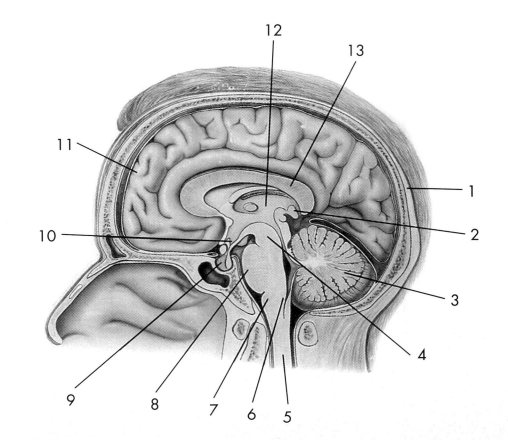

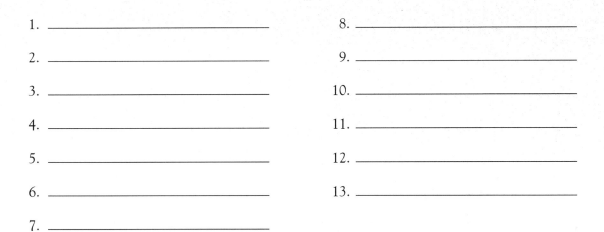

1. _____	8. _____
2. _____	9. _____
3. _____	10. _____
4. _____	11. _____
5. _____	12. _____
6. _____	13. _____
7. _____	

Neuron Pathways

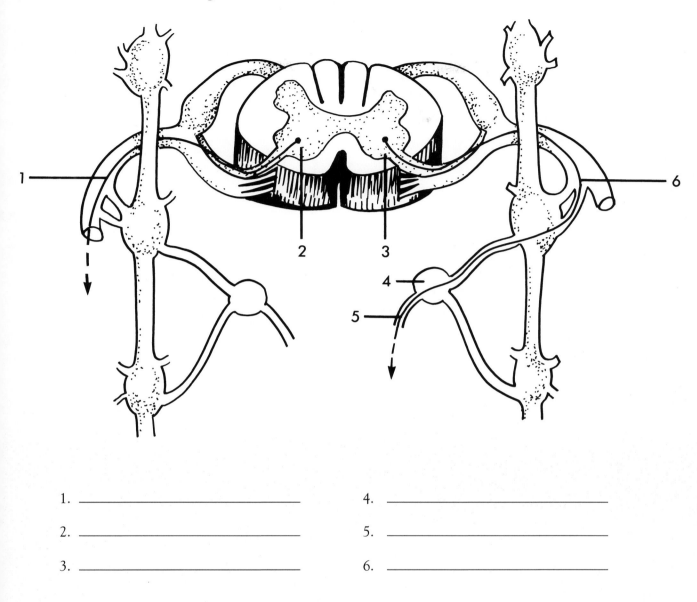

1. _____   4. _____

2. _____   5. _____

3. _____   6. _____

CHAPTER **8**

The Senses

Consider this scene for a moment. You are walking along a beautiful beach watching the sunset. You notice the various hues and are amazed at the multitude of shades that cover the sky. The waves are indeed melodious as they splash along the shore, and you wiggle your feet with delight as you sense the warm, soft sand trickling between your toes. You sip on a soda and then inhale the fresh salt air as you continue your stroll along the shore. It is a memorable scene, but one that would not be possible without the assistance of your sense organs. The sense organs pick up messages that are sent over nerve pathways to specialized areas in the brain for interpretation. They make communication with and enjoyment of the environment possible. The visual, auditory, tactile, olfactory, and gustatory sense organs not only protect us from danger but also add an important dimension to our daily pleasures of life.

Your study of this chapter will give you an understanding of another one of the systems necessary for homeostasis and survival.

TOPICS FOR REVIEW

Before progressing to Chapter 9, you should review the classification of sense organs and the process for converting a stimulus into a sensation. Your study should also include an understanding of the special sense organs and the general sense organs.

CLASSIFICATION OF SENSE ORGANS
CONVERTING A STIMULUS INTO A SENSATION
GENERAL SENSE ORGANS

Match the term on the left with the proper selection on the right.

_____ 1. Special sense organ

_____ 2. General sense organ

_____ 3. Nose

_____ 4. Krause's end-bulbs

_____ 5. Taste buds

A. Olfactory cells

B. Meissner's corpuscles

C. Chemoreceptor

D. Eye

E. Touch

▶ *If you have had difficulty with this section, review pages 204-206.*

SPECIAL SENSE ORGANS

Eye

Circle the correct answer.

6. The "white" of the eye is more commonly called the:
   A. Choroid
   B. Cornea
   C. Sclera
   D. Retina
   E. None of the above

7. The "colored" part of the eye is known as the:
   A. Retina
   B. Cornea
   C. Pupil
   D. Sclera
   E. Iris

8. The transparent portion of the sclera, referred to as the "window" of the eye, is the:
   A. Retina
   B. Cornea
   C. Pupil
   D. Iris

9. The mucous membrane that covers the front of the eye is called the:
   A. Cornea
   B. Choroid
   C. Conjunctiva
   D. Ciliary body
   E. None of the above

10. The structure that can contract or dilate to allow more or less light to enter the eye is the:
    A. Lens
    B. Choroid
    C. Retina
    D. Cornea
    E. Iris
11. When the eye is looking at objects far in the distance, the lens is _____ and the ciliary muscle is _____.
    A. Rounded, contracted
    B. Rounded, relaxed
    C. Slightly rounded, contracted
    D. Slightly curved, relaxed
    E. None of the above
12. The lens of the eye is held in place by the:
    A. Ciliary muscle
    B. Aqueous humor
    C. Vitreous humor
    D. Cornea
13. When the lens loses its elasticity and can no longer bring near objects into focus, the condition is known as:
    A. Glaucoma
    B. Presbyopia
    C. Astigmatism
    D. Strabismus
14. The fluid in front of the lens that is constantly being formed, drained, and replaced in the anterior chamber is the:
    A. Vitreous humor
    B. Protoplasm
    C. Aqueous humor
    D. Conjunctiva
15. If drainage of the aqueous humor is blocked, the internal pressure within the eye will increase and a condition known as _____ could occur.
    A. Presbyopia
    B. Glaucoma
    C. Color blindness
    D. Cataracts
16. The rods and cones are the photoreceptor cells and are located on the:
    A. Sclera
    B. Cornea
    C. Choroid
    D. Retina
17. The area that contains the greatest concentration of cones on the retina is the:
    A. Fovea centralis
    B. Retinal artery
    C. Ciliary body
    D. Optic disc

18. If our eyes are abnormally elongated, the image focuses in front of the retina and a condition known as _____ occurs.
    A. Hyperopia
    B. Cataracts
    C. Night blindness
    D. Myopia

 If you have had difficulty with this section, review pages 204-211.

Ear

Select the correct term from the choices given and write its letter in the answer blank.

| A. External ear | B. Middle ear | C. Inner ear |

_____ 19. Malleus
_____ 20. Perilymph
_____ 21. Incus
_____ 22. Ceruminous glands
_____ 23. Cochlea
_____ 24. Auditory canal
_____ 25. Semicircular canals
_____ 26. Stapes
_____ 27. Eustachian tube
_____ 28. Organ of Corti

Fill in the blanks.

29. The external ear has two parts: the _____ and the _____
    _____ _____.
30. Another name for the tympanic membrane is the _____.
31. The bones of the middle ear are collectively referred to as the _____.
32. The stapes presses against a membrane that covers a small opening called the
    _____ _____.
33. A middle ear infection is called _____ _____.
34. The _____ is located adjacent to the oval window between the semicircular canals and the cochlea.
35. Located within the semicircular canals and the vestibule are _____ for balance and equilibrium.
36. The sensory cells in the _____ _____ are stimulated when movement of the head causes the endolymph to move.

 If you have had difficulty with this section, review pages 213-214.

TASTE RECEPTORS
SMELL RECEPTORS

Circle the correct answer.

37. Structures known as (papillae or olfactory) cells are found on the tongue.
38. Nerve impulses generated by stimulation of taste buds travel primarily through two (cranial or spinal) nerves.
39. To be detected by olfactory receptors, chemicals must be dissolved in the watery (mucus or plasma) that lines the nasal cavity.
40. The pathways taken by olfactory nerve impulses and the areas where these impulses are interpreted are closely associated with areas of the brain important in (hearing or memory).
41. (Chemoreceptor or mechanoreceptor) is the term used to describe the type of receptors that generate nervous impulses resulting in the sense of taste or smell.

▶ *If you have had difficulty with this section, review pages 214-218.*

UNSCRAMBLE THE WORDS

42. C A L R I E U

43. R A E C L S

44. L A P I L A E P

45. C T V N U C N O I A J

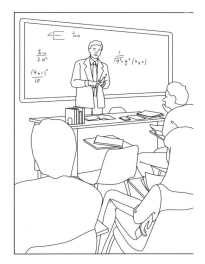

Take the circled letters, unscramble them, and fill in the statement.

What Mr. Tuttle liked best about his classroom.

46.

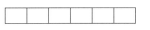

APPLYING WHAT YOU KNOW

47. Mr. Nay was an avid swimmer and competed regularly in his age group. He had to withdraw from the last competition due to an infection of his ear. Antibiotics and analgesics were prescribed by the doctor. What is the medical term for his condition?

Chapter 8: The Senses   101

48. Mrs. Metheny loved the outdoors and spent a great deal of her spare time basking in the sun on the beach. Her physician suggested that she begin wearing sunglasses regularly when he noticed milky spots beginning to appear on Mrs. Metheny's lenses. What condition was Mrs. Metheny's physician trying to prevent?

_____

49. Amanda repeatedly became ill with throat infections during her first few years of school. Lately, however, she has noticed that whenever she has a throat infection, her ears become very sore also. What might be the cause of this additional problem?

_____

50. Julius was hit in the nose with a baseball during practice. His sense of smell was temporarily gone. What nerve receptors were damaged during the injury?

_____

51. WORD FIND

Can you find 19 terms from this chapter? Words may be spelled top to bottom, bottom to top, right to left, left to right, or diagonally.

```
M E C H A N O R E C E P T O R
H R A T B Q I R T B N H M A E
P F T Y R O T C A F L O X R C
G U A Y I N A I H C A T S U E
G P R A C E R U M E N O P X P
I E A I P O Y B S E R P K D T
W L C P L Y N E Y K E I T O O
C Q T O I B R J B S F G L M R
Z U S R C L E O U J R M N N S
F D M E O H L Q T N A E Y I S
H I D P N D L A M A C N X S Z
A M L Y E S S E E D T T M Z H
D D M H S F E X A Y I S I I A
J C G N J T I S L P O G U V J
P H G Y A K H S U C N I S G A
```

Cataracts	Gustatory	Presbyopia
Cerumen	Hyperopia	Receptors
Cochlea	Incus	Refraction
Cones	Mechanoreceptor	Rods
Conjunctiva	Olfactory	Senses
Eustachian	Papillae	
Eye	Photopigment	

THE SENSES

Fill in the crossword puzzle.

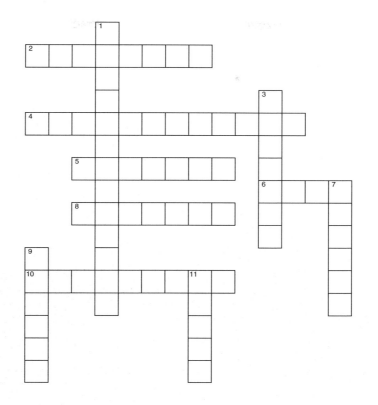

Across

2. Bones of the middle ear
4. Located in anterior cavity in front of lens (two words)
5. External ear
6. Transparent body behind pupil
8. Front part of this coat is the ciliary muscle and iris
10. Membranous labyrinth is filled with this fluid

Down

1. Located in posterior cavity (two words)
3. Organ of Corti located here
7. White of the eye
9. Innermost layer of the eye
11. Hole in the center of the iris

CHECK YOUR KNOWLEDGE
Multiple Choice

Circle the correct answer.

1. Where are the specialized mechanoreceptors of hearing and balance located?
   A. Inner ear
   B. Malleus
   C. Helix
   D. All of the above

2. The organ of Corti is the sense organ of what sense?
   A. Sight
   B. Hearing
   C. Pressure
   D. Taste

3. Where are taste sensations interpreted?
   A. Cerebral cortex
   B. Area of stimulation
   C. Nasal cavity
   D. None of the above

4. A surgical technique to treat myopia without the use of glasses or contacts is called:
   A. Presbyopia
   B. Removal of cataracts
   C. Radial keratotomy
   D. None of the above

5. Which of the following statements about the cornea is *true*?
   A. It is a mucous membrane.
   B. It is called the "window of the eye."
   C. It lies behind the iris.
   D. All of the above

6. Which of the following are general sense organs?
   A. Gustatory receptors
   B. Pacinian corpuscles
   C. Olfactory receptors
   D. All of the above

7. The retina contains microscopic receptor cells called:
   A. Mechanoreceptors
   B. Chemoreceptors
   C. Olfactory receptors
   D. Rods and cones

8. Which two involuntary muscles make up the front part of the eye?
   A. Malleus and incus
   B. Iris and ciliary muscle
   C. Retina and pacinian muscle
   D. Sclera and iris

9. Which of the following statements about gustatory sense organs is *true*?
    A. They are called taste buds.
    B. They are innervated by cranial nerves VII and IX.
    C. They work together with the olfactory senses.
    D. All of the above
10. The external ear consists of the:
    A. Auricle and auditory canal
    B. Labyrinth
    C. Corti and cochlea
    D. None of the above

True or False

Indicate whether the following statements are true (T) or false (F).

_____ 11. The tympanic membrane separates the middle ear from the external ear.

_____ 12. Glaucoma may result from a blockage of the flow of the vitreous humor.

_____ 13. With the condition of presbyopia, the eye lens loses its elasticity.

_____ 14. The crista ampullaris is located in the nasal cavity.

_____ 15. Myopia occurs when images are focused in front of the retina rather than on it.

_____ 16. Light enters through the pupil, and the size of the pupil is regulated by the iris.

_____ 17. The retina is the innermost layer of the eye. It contains the structures called rods.

_____ 18. The sclera is commonly called the "white of the eye."

_____ 19. The olfactory receptors are chemical receptors.

_____ 20. The organ of Corti contains mechanoreceptors.

Eye

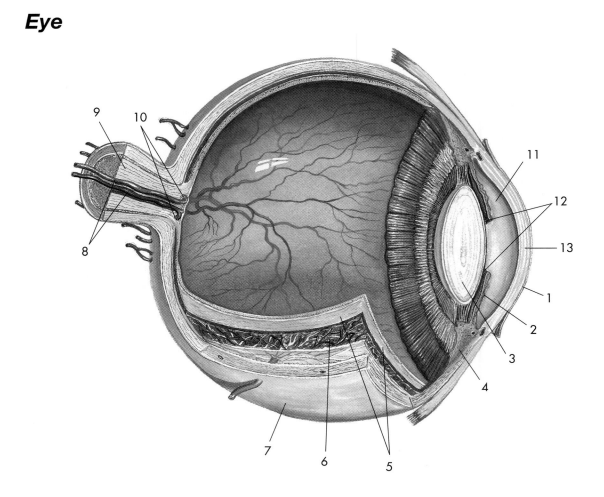

1. _____

2. _____

3. _____

4. _____

5. _____

6. _____

7. _____

8. _____

9. _____

10. _____

11. _____

12. _____

13. _____

Ear

1. _____

2. _____

3. _____

4. _____

5. _____

6. _____

7. _____

8. _____

9. _____

10. _____

11. _____

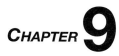

The Endocrine System

The endocrine system has often been compared to a fine concert symphony. When all instruments are playing properly, the sound is melodious. If one instrument plays too loud or too soft, however, it affects the overall quality of the entire performance.

The endocrine system is a ductless system that releases hormones into the bloodstream to help regulate body functions. The pituitary gland may be considered the conductor of the orchestra, as it stimulates many of the endocrine glands to secrete their powerful hormones. All hormones, whether stimulated in this manner or by other control mechanisms, are interdependent. A change in the level of one hormone may affect the level of many other hormones.

In addition to the endocrine glands, prostaglandins ("tissue hormones") are powerful substances similar to hormones that have been found in a variety of body tissues. These hormones are often produced in a tissue and diffuse only a short distance to act on cells within that area. Prostaglandins influence respiration, blood pressure, gastrointestinal secretions, and the reproductive system, and they may some day play an important role in the treatment of diseases such as hypertension, asthma, and ulcers.

The endocrine system is a system of communication and control. It differs from the nervous system in that hormones provide a slower, longer-lasting effect than do nerve stimuli and responses. Your understanding of the "system of hormones" will alert you to the mechanisms of our emotions, our responses to stress, our growth, our chemical balances, and many other of our body functions.

TOPICS FOR REVIEW

Before progressing to Chapter 10, you should be able to identify and locate the primary endocrine glands of the body. Your understanding should include the hormones that are produced by these glands and the method by which these secretions are regulated. Your study will conclude with the pathological conditions that result from the malfunctioning of this system.

MECHANISMS OF HORMONE ACTION
REGULATION OF HORMONE SECRETION
PROSTAGLANDINS

Match the term on the left with the proper selection on the right.

Group A

_____	1. Pituitary	A. Pelvic cavity
_____	2. Parathyroids	B. Mediastinum
_____	3. Adrenals	C. Neck
_____	4. Ovaries	D. Cranial cavity
_____	5. Thymus	E. Abdominal cavity

Group B

_____	6. Negative feedback	A. Explanation for hormone organ recognition
_____	7. Tissue hormones	B. Respond to a particular hormone
_____	8. Second messenger hypothesis	C. Prostaglandins
_____	9. Exocrine glands	D. Discharge secretions into ducts
_____	10. Target organ cells	E. Specialized homeostatic mechanism that regulates release of hormones

Fill in the blanks.

The (11) _____ _____ hypothesis is a theory that attempts to

explain why hormones cause specific effects in target organs but do not (12) _____

or act on other organs of the body. Protein hormones serve as (13) _____

_____, providing communication between endocrine glands and

(14) _____ _____. The second messenger

(15) _____ _____ provides communication within a hormone's

(16) _____ _____. (17) The study of the important roles of the

_____ _____ and _____

_____ in second messenger systems resulted in Nobel Prizes.

▶ *If you have had difficulty with this section, review pages 225-231.*

PITUITARY GLAND
HYPOTHALAMUS

Circle the correct answer.

18. The pituitary gland lies in the _____ bone.
    A. Ethmoid
    B. Sphenoid
    C. Temporal
    D. Frontal
    E. Occipital

19. Which one of the following structures would *not* be stimulated by a tropic hormone from the anterior pituitary?
    A. Ovaries
    B. Testes
    C. Thyroid
    D. Adrenals
    E. Uterus

20. Which one of the following is *not* a function of FSH?
    A. Stimulates the growth of follicles
    B. Stimulates the production of estrogens
    C. Stimulates the growth of seminiferous tubules
    D. Stimulates the interstitial cells of the testes

21. Which one of the following is *not* a function of LH?
    A. Stimulates the maturation of a developing follicle
    B. Stimulates the production of estrogens
    C. Stimulates the formation of a corpus luteum
    D. Stimulates sperm cells to mature in the male
    E. Causes ovulation

22. Which one of the following is *not* a function of GH?
    A. Increases glucose catabolism
    B. Increases fat catabolism
    C. Speeds up the movement of amino acids into cells from the bloodstream
    D. All of the above are functions of GH

23. Which one of the following hormones is *not* released by the anterior pituitary gland?
    A. ACT
    B. TSH
    C. ADH
    D. FSH
    E. LH

24. Which one of the following is *not* a function of prolactin?
    A. Stimulates breast development during pregnancy
    B. Stimulates milk secretion after delivery
    C. Causes the release of milk from glandular cells of the breast
    D. All of the above are functions of prolactin
25. The anterior pituitary gland:
    A. Secretes eight major hormones
    B. Secretes tropic hormones that stimulate other endocrine glands to grow and secrete
    C. Secretes ADH
    D. Secretes oxytocin
26. TSH acts on the:
    A. Thyroid
    B. Thymus
    C. Pineal
    D. Testes
27. ACTH stimulates the:
    A. Adrenal cortex
    B. Adrenal medulla
    C. Hypothalamus
    D. Ovaries
28. Which hormone is secreted by the posterior pituitary gland?
    A. MSH
    B. LH
    C. GH
    D. ADH
29. ADH serves the body by:
    A. Initiating labor
    B. Accelerating water reabsorption from urine into the blood
    C. Stimulating the pineal gland
    D. Regulating the calcium/phosphorus levels in the blood
30. What disease is caused by hyposecretion of the ADH?
    A. Diabetes insipidus
    B. Diabetes mellitus
    C. Acromegaly
    D. Myxedema
31. The actual production of ADH and oxytocin takes place in which area?
    A. Anterior pituitary
    B. Posterior pituitary
    C. Hypothalamus
    D. Pineal
32. Inhibiting hormones are produced by the:
    A. Anterior pituitary
    B. Posterior pituitary
    C. Hypothalamus
    D. Pineal

Select the correct term from the choices given and write the letter in the answer blank.

     A. Anterior pituitary   B. Posterior pituitary   C. Hypothalamus

_____ 33. Adenohypophysis

_____ 34. Neurohypophysis

_____ 35. Induced labor

_____ 36. Appetite

_____ 37. Acromegaly

_____ 38. Body temperature

_____ 39. Sex hormones

_____ 40. Tropic hormones

_____ 41. Gigantism

_____ 42. Releasing hormones

 If you have had difficulty with this section, review pages 231-235.

THYROID GLAND
PARATHYROID GLANDS

Circle the correct answer.

43. The thyroid gland lies (above or below) the larynx.
44. The thyroid gland secretes (calcitonin or glucagon).
45. For thyroxine to be produced in adequate amounts, the diet must contain sufficient (calcium or iodine).
46. Most endocrine glands (do or do not) store their hormones.
47. Colloid is a storage medium for the (thyroid or parathyroid) hormone.
48. Calcitonin (increases or decreases) the concentration of calcium in the blood.
49. Simple goiter results from (hyperthyroidism or hypothyroidism).
50. Hyposecretion of thyroid hormones during the formative years leads to (cretinism or myxedema).
51. The parathyroid glands secrete the hormone (PTH or PTA).
52. Parathyroid hormone tends to (increase or decrease) the concentration of calcium in the blood.

If you have had difficulty with this section, review pages 235-237.

ADRENAL GLANDS

Fill in the blanks.

53. The adrenal gland is actually two separate endocrine glands, the _____ _____ and the _____ _____.
54. Hormones secreted by the adrenal cortex are known as _____.
55. The outer zone of the adrenal cortex secretes _____.
56. The middle zone secretes _____.
57. The innermost zone secretes _____ _____.

58. Glucocorticoids act in several ways to increase _____.

59. Glucocorticoids also play an essential part in maintaining _____
_____.

60. The adrenal medulla secretes the hormones _____ and
_____.

61. The adrenal medulla may help the body resist _____.

62. Deficiency or hyposecretion of adrenal cortex hormones results in a condition called
_____ _____.

Select the correct term from the choices given and write the letter in the answer blank.

     A. Adrenal cortex   B. Adrenal medulla

_____ 63. Mineralocorticoids

_____ 64. Anti-immunity

_____ 65. Adrenaline

_____ 66. Cushing's syndrome

_____ 67. "Fight or flight" syndrome

_____ 68. Aldosterone

_____ 69. Androgens

▶ *If you have had difficulty with this section, review pages 236-241.*

PANCREATIC ISLETS
SEX GLANDS
THYMUS
PLACENTA
PINEAL GLAND

Circle the term that does not belong.

70. Alpha cells	Glucagon	Beta cells	Glycogenolysis
71. Insulin	Glucagon	Beta cells	Diabetes mellitus
72. Estrogens	Progesterone	Corpus luteum	Thymosin
73. Chorion	Interstitial cells	Testosterone	Semen
74. Immune system	Mediastinum	Aldosterone	Thymosin
75. Pregnancy	ACTH	Estrogen	Chorion
76. Melatonin	Menstruation	"Third eye"	Semen

Match the term on the left with the proper selection on the right.

Group A

———— 77. Alpha cells

———— 78. Beta cells

———— 79. Corpus luteum

———— 80. Interstitial cells

———— 81. Ovarian follicles

A. Estrogen
B. Progesterone
C. Insulin
D. Testosterone
E. Glucagon

Group B

———— 82. Placenta

———— 83. Pineal

———— 84. Heart atria

———— 85. Testes

———— 86. Thymus

A. Melatonin
B. ANH
C. Testosterone
D. Thymosin
E. Chorionic gonadotropins

 If you have had difficulty with this section, review pages 242-246.

UNSCRAMBLE THE WORDS

87. ROODIITSCC

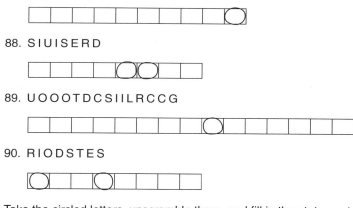

88. SIUISERD

89. UOOOTDCSIILRCCG

90. RIODSTES

Take the circled letters, unscramble them, and fill in the statement.

Why Billy didn't like to take exams.

91.

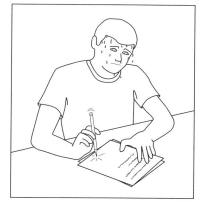

APPLYING WHAT YOU KNOW

92. Mrs. Fortner made a routine visit to her physician last week. When the laboratory results came back, the report indicated a high level of chorionic gonadotropin in her urine. What did this mean to Mrs. Fortner?

_____

93. Mrs. Wilcox noticed that her daughter was beginning to take on the secondary sex characteristics of a male. The pediatrician diagnosed the condition as a tumor of an endocrine gland. Where specifically was the tumor located?

_____

_____

94. Mrs. Hart was pregnant and was 2 weeks past her due date. Her doctor suggested that she enter the hospital and said he would induce labor. What hormone will he give Mrs. Hart?

_____

95. WORD FIND

Can you find 16 terms from this chapter? Words may be spelled top to bottom, bottom to top, right to left, left to right, or diagonally.

```
S  S  I  S  E  R  U  I  D  M  E  S  I  T  W
N  D  N  X  E  B  A  M  E  D  E  X  Y  M  I
I  I  G  O  N  R  S  G  X  T  I  I  Y  V  B
D  O  M  S  I  N  I  T  E  R  C  C  U  Q  D
N  C  X  S  R  T  N  B  O  T  V  M  Y  O  M
A  I  M  E  C  L  A  C  R  E  P  Y  H  I  X
L  T  Y  R  O  I  E  Z  Q  R  T  J  V  K  F
G  R  E  T  D  P  S  N  I  L  D  J  M  X  N
A  O  O  S  N  I  D  K  I  N  K  S  P  P  O
T  C  P  R  E  T  I  O  G  R  I  F  M  X  G
S  L  M  H  Y  P  O  G  L  Y  C  E  M  I  A
O  A  J  L  H  O  R  M  O  N  E  O  T  G  C
R  C  E  L  T  S  E  L  C  N  P  N  X  U  U
P  I  O  S  W  R  T  X  C  G  U  L  O  E  L
G  G  V  Y  H  M  S  H  Y  K  A  K  N  Q  G
```

Corticoids	Glucagon	Myxedema
Cretinism	Goiter	Prostaglandins
Diabetes	Hormone	Steroids
Diuresis	Hypercalcemia	Stress
Endocrine	Hypoglycemia	
Exocrine	Luteinization	

DID YOU KNOW?

The total daily output of the pituitary gland is less than 1/1,000,000 of a gram, yet this small amount is responsible for stimulating the majority of all endocrine functions.

THE ENDOCRINE SYSTEM

Fill in the crossword puzzle.

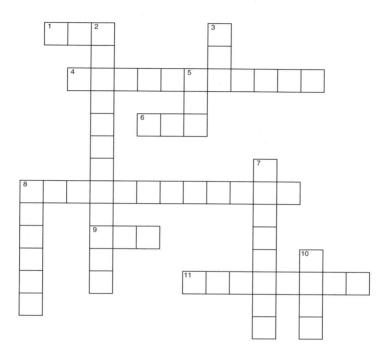

Across

1. Secreted by cells in the walls of the heart's atria
4. Adrenal medulla
6. Estrogens
8. Converts amino acids into glucose
9. Melanin
11. Labor

Down

2. Hypersecretion of insulin
3. Antagonist to diuresis
5. Increases calcium concentration
7. Hyposecretion of Islands of Langerhans (one word)
8. Hyposecretion of thyroid
10. Adrenal cortex

CHECK YOUR KNOWLEDGE
Multiple Choice

Circle the correct answer.

1. What does the outer zone of the adrenal cortex secrete?
   A. Mineralocorticoids
   B. Sex hormones
   C. Glucocorticoids
   D. Epinephrine

2. From what condition does diabetes insipidus result?
   A. Low insulin levels
   B. High glucagon levels
   C. Low antidiuretic hormone levels
   D. High steroid levels

3. Which of the following statements about a young child whose growth is stunted, whose metabolism is low, whose sexual development is delayed, and whose mental development is retarded is *true*?
   A. The child suffers from cretinism.
   B. The child has an underactive thyroid.
   C. The child could suffer from a pituitary disorder.
   D. All of the above

4. What can result when too much growth hormone is produced by the pituitary gland?
   A. Hyperglycemia
   B. A pituitary giant
   C. Both A and B
   D. None of the above

5. Which of the following glands is *not* regulated by the pituitary?
   A. Thyroid
   B. Ovaries
   C. Adrenals
   D. Thymus

6. Which of the following statements about antidiuretic hormone is *true*?
   A. It is released by the posterior lobe of the pituitary.
   B. It causes diabetes insipidus when produced in insufficient amounts.
   C. It decreases urine volume.
   D. All of the above

7. What controls the development of the body's immune system?
   A. Pituitary
   B. Thymus
   C. Pineal body
   D. Thyroid
8. Administration of what would best treat a person suffering from severe allergies?
   A. Gonadocorticoids
   B. Glucagon
   C. Mineralocorticoids
   D. Glucocorticoids
9. What endocrine gland is composed of cell clusters called the islets of Langerhans?
   A. Adrenals
   B. Thyroid
   C. Pituitary
   D. Pancreas
10. Which of the following statements concerning prostaglandins is *true*?
    A. They control activities of widely separated organs.
    B. They can be called tissue hormones.
    C. They diffuse over long distances to act on cells.
    D. All of the above

Matching

Select the most appropriate answer from column B for each item in column A. There is only one correct answer for each item.

Column A	Column B
_____ 11. Goiter	A. Glucocorticoid hormones
_____ 12. Ovulation	B. Antidiuretic hormone
_____ 13. Diabetes mellitus	C. Calcitonin
_____ 14. Lactation	D. Oxytocin
_____ 15. Diabetes insipidus	E. Growth hormone
_____ 16. Chorionic gonadotropins	F. Placenta
_____ 17. Cushing's syndrome	G. Luteinizing hormone
_____ 18. Labor	H. Insulin
_____ 19. Acromegaly	I. Prolactin
_____ 20. Hypercalcemia	J. Thyroid hormones

Endocrine Glands

1. _____

2. _____

3. _____

4. _____

5. _____

6. _____

7. _____

8. _____

9. _____

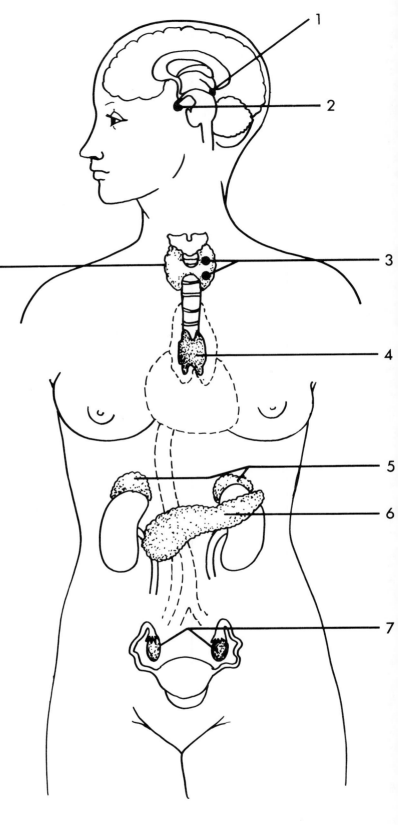

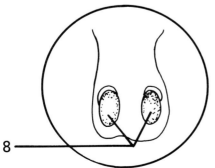

Blood, the river of life, is the body's primary means of transportation. Although it is the respiratory system that provides oxygen for the body, the digestive system that provides nutrients, and the urinary system that eliminates wastes, none of these functions could be provided for the individual cells without the blood. In less than one minute, a drop of blood will complete a trip through the entire body, distributing nutrients and collecting the wastes of metabolism.

Blood is divided into plasma (the liquid portion of blood) and the formed elements (the blood cells). There are three types of blood cells: red blood cells, white blood cells, and platelets. Together these cells and plasma provide a means of transportation that delivers the body's daily necessities.

Although the red blood cells in all of us are of a similar shape, we have different blood types. Blood types are identified by the presence of certain antigens in the red blood cells. Every person's blood belongs to one of four main blood groups: A, B, AB, or O. Any one of the four groups or "types" may or may not have the specific antigen called the Rh factor present in the red blood cells. If an individual has the Rh factor present in his or her blood, the blood is Rh positive. If this factor is missing, the blood is Rh negative. Approximately, 85% of the population have the Rh factor (Rh positive), and 15% do not have the Rh factor (Rh negative).

Your understanding of this chapter will be necessary to prepare a proper foundation for the circulatory system.

TOPICS FOR REVIEW

Before progressing to Chapter 11, you should have an understanding of the structure and function of blood plasma and cells. Your review should also include a knowledge of blood types and Rh factors.

BLOOD COMPOSITION

Circle the correct answer.

1. Which one of the following substances is not a part of the plasma?
   A. Hormones
   B. Salts
   C. Nutrients
   D. Wastes
   E. All of the above are part of the plasma

2. The normal volume of blood in an adult is about:
   A. 2-3 pints
   B. 2-3 quarts
   C. 2-3 gallons
   D. 4-6 liters

3. Another name for red blood cells is:
   A. Leukocytes
   B. Thrombocytes
   C. Platelets
   D. Erythrocytes

4. Another name for white blood cells is:
   A. Erythrocytes
   B. Leukocytes
   C. Thrombocytes
   D. Platelets

5. Another name for platelets is:
   A. Neutrophils
   B. Eosinophils
   C. Thrombocytes
   D. Erythrocytes

6. Pernicious anemia is caused by:
   A. A lack of vitamin B_{12}
   B. Hemorrhage
   C. Radiation
   D. Bleeding ulcers

7. The laboratory test called hematocrit tells the physician:
   A. The volume of white cells in a blood sample
   B. The volume of red cells in a blood sample
   C. The volume of platelets in a blood sample
   D. The volume of plasma in a blood sample

8. An example of a nongranular leukocyte is a/an:
   A. Platelet
   B. Erythrocyte
   C. Eosinophil
   D. Monocyte

9. An abnormally high white blood cell count is known as:
   A. Leukemia
   B. Leukopenia
   C. Leukocytosis
   D. Anemia
10. A critical component of hemoglobin is:
    A. Potassium
    B. Calcium
    C. Vitamin K
    D. Iron
11. Sickle cell anemia is caused by:
    A. The production of an abnormal type of hemoglobin
    B. The production of excessive neutrophils
    C. The production of excessive platelets
    D. The production of abnormal leukocytes
12. The practice of using blood transfusions to increase oxygen delivery to muscles during athletic events is called:
    A. Blood antigen
    B. Blood doping
    C. Blood agglutination
    D. Blood proofing
13. The term used to describe the condition of a circulating blood clot is:
    A. Thrombosis
    B. Embolism
    C. Hemoglobin
    D. Platelet
14. Which one of the following types of cells is *not* a granular leukocyte?
    A. Neutrophil
    B. Lymphocyte
    C. Basophil
    D. Eosinophil
15. If a blood cell has no nucleus and is shaped like a biconcave disc, then the cell most likely is a/an:
    A. Platelet
    B. Lymphocyte
    C. Basophil
    D. Eosinophil
    E. Red blood cell
16. Red bone marrow forms all kinds of blood cells, *except* some:
    A. Platelets
    B. Lymphocytes
    C. Red blood cells
    D. Neutrophils

17. Myeloid tissue is found in all but which one of the following locations?
   A. Sternum
   B. Ribs
   C. Wrist bones
   D. Hip bones
   E. Cranial bones
18. Lymphatic tissue is found in all but which of the following locations?
   A. Lymph nodes
   B. Thymus
   C. Spleen
   D. All of the above contain lymphatic tissue
19. The "buffy coat" layer in a hematocrit tube contains:
   A. Red blood cells and platelets
   B. Plasma only
   C. Platelets only
   D. White blood cells and platelets
   E. None of the above
20. The hematocrit value for red blood cells is:
   A. 75%
   B. 60%
   C. 50%
   D. 45%
   E. 35%
21. An unusually low white blood cell count would be termed:
   A. Leukemia
   B. Leukopenia
   C. Leukocytosis
   D. Anemia
   E. None of the above
22. Most of the oxygen transported in the blood is carried by:
   A. Platelets
   B. Plasma
   C. Basophils
   D. Red blood cells
   E. None of the above
23. The most numerous of the phagocytes are the:
   A. Lymphocytes
   B. Neutrophils
   C. Basophils
   D. Eosinophils
   E. Monocytes

24. Which one of the following types of cells is *not* phagocytic?
    A. Neutrophils
    B. Eosinophils
    C. Lymphocytes
    D. Monocytes
    E. All of the above are phagocytic cells
25. Which of the following cell types functions in the immune process?
    A. Neutrophils
    B. Lymphocytes
    C. Monocytes
    D. Basophils
    E. Reticuloendothelial cells
26. The organ that manufactures prothrombin is the:
    A. Liver
    B. Pancreas
    C. Thymus
    D. Kidney
    E. Spleen
27. Which one of the following vitamins acts to accelerate blood clotting?
    A. A
    B. B
    C. C
    D. D
    E. K

▶ *If you have had difficulty with this section, review pages 256-265.*

BLOOD TYPES
RH FACTOR

28. Fill in the missing areas of the chart.

Blood Type	Antigen Present in RBCs	Antibody Present in Plasma
A	_____	Anti-B
B	B	_____
AB	_____	None
O	None	_____

Fill in the blanks

29. An _____ is a substance that can activate the immune system to make antibodies.

30. An _____ is a substance made by the body in response to stimulation by an antigen.

31. Many antibodies react with their antigens to clump or _____ them.

32. If a baby is born to an Rh negative mother and Rh positive father, it may develop the disease _____ _____.

33. The term "Rh" is used because the antigen was first discovered in the blood of _____ _____.

34. _____ stops an Rh negative mother from forming anti-Rh antibodies and thus prevents the possibility of harm to her next Rh positive baby.

35. Blood type _____ has been called the universal recipient.

▶ *If you have had difficulty with this section, review pages 262-265.*

APPLYING WHAT YOU KNOW

36. Mrs. Payne's blood type is O positive. Her husband's type is O negative. Her newborn baby's blood type is O negative. Is there any need for concern with this combination?

   _____

37. After Mrs. Freund's baby was born, the doctor applied a gauze dressing to the umbilical cord for a short time. He also gave the baby a dose of vitamin K. Why did the doctor perform these two procedures?

   _____

38. WORD FIND

Can you find 24 terms from this chapter? Words may be spelled top to bottom, bottom to top, right to left, left to right, or diagonally.

```
H S H K L S U L O B M E A E S
K E E V M Z H E P A R I N D N
D T M F A C T O R Y E T I Q P
O Y A O H N B A T Q Y A R A R
N C T J G W E H N P N L B U D
O O O S Q L R M E T I S I P M
R K C E M O O N I H I Q F W W
H U R T C N I B P A S G Z T G
E E I Y O B O O I V E W E T X
S L T C M D S E C N R T U N R
U E Y O Y A I M E K U E L Y S
S T R G B S T H R O M B U S Q
E H Z A M S A L P N D Z P O N
T E N H F P D A P M E E I B W
E W B P H K B O N C K W X V J
```

AIDS   Factor   Phagocytes
Anemia   Fibrin   Plasma
Antibody   Hematocrit   Recipient
Antigen   Hemoglobin   Rhesus
Basophil   Heparin   Serum
Donor   Leukemia   Thrombin
Embolus   Leukocytes   Thrombus
Erythrocytes   Monocyte   Type

DID YOU KNOW?

Blood products are good for approximately 21 days, whereas fresh frozen plasma is good for at least 6 months.

BLOOD

Fill in the crossword puzzle.

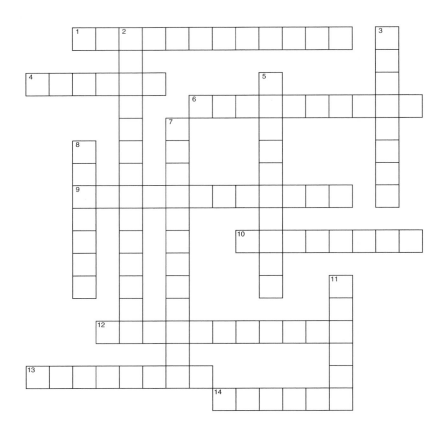

Across

1. Abnormally high WBC count
4. Final stage of clotting process
6. Oxygen-carrying mechanism of blood
9. To engulf and digest microbes
10. Stationary blood clot
12. RBC
13. Circulating blood clot
14. Liquid portion of the blood

Down

2. Type O (two words)
3. Substances that stimulate the body to make antibodies
5. Type of leukocyte
7. Platelets
8. Prevents the clotting of blood
11. Inability of the blood to carry sufficient oxygen

CHECK YOUR KNOWLEDGE

Multiple Choice

Circle the correct answer.

1. Which of the following statements is *false*?
   A. Sickle cell anemia is caused by a genetic defect.
   B. Leukemia is characterized by a low number of WBCs.
   C. Polycythemia is characterized by an abnormally high number of erythrocytes.
   D. Pernicious anemia is caused by a lack of vitamin B_{12}.
2. Deficiency in the number or function of erythrocytes is called:
   A. Leukemia
   B. Anemia
   C. Polycythemia
   D. Leukopenia
3. Which of the following statements do *not* describe a characteristic of leukocytes?
   A. They are disk-shaped cells that do not contain a nucleus.
   B. They have the ability to fight infection.
   C. They provide defense against certain parasites.
   D. They provide immune defense.
4. Which of the following substances is *not* found in serum?
   A. Clotting factors
   B. Water
   C. Hormones
   D. All of the above substances are found in serum
5. Which of the following substances is *not* found in blood plasma?
   A. Water
   B. Oxygen
   C. Hormones
   D. None of the above
6. An allergic reaction may increase the number of:
   A. Eosinophils
   B. Neutrophils
   C. Lymphocytes
   D. Monocytes
7. What is a blood clot that is moving through the body called?
   A. Embolism
   B. Fibrosis
   C. Heparin
   D. Thrombosis
8. When could difficulty with the Rh blood factor arise?
   A. When an Rh negative man and woman produce a child.
   B. When an Rh positive man and woman produce a child.
   C. When an Rh positive woman and an Rh negative man produce a child.
   D. When an Rh negative woman and an Rh positive man produce a child.

9. What is the primary function of hemoglobin?
    A. To fight infection
    B. To cause blood to clot
    C. To carry oxygen
    D. To transport hormones
10. Which of the following steps is *not* involved in blood clot formation?
    A. A blood vessel is injured and platelet factors are formed.
    B. Thrombin is converted into prothrombin.
    C. Fibrinogen is converted into fibrin.
    D. All of the above are involved in blood clot formation

Matching

Select the most appropriate answer from column B for each item in column A. There is only one correct answer for each item.

Column A	Column B
_____ 11. Lymphocytes	A. Heparin
_____ 12. Erythrocytes	B. Contains anti-A and anti-B antibodies
_____ 13. Type AB	C. Clotting
_____ 14. Basophils	D. Immunity
_____ 15. Leukemia	E. Erythroblastosis fetalis
_____ 16. Platelets	F. Anemia
_____ 17. Type O	G. Cancer
_____ 18. Rh factor	H. Contains A and B antigens
_____ 19. Red bone marrow	I. Myeloid tissue
_____ 20. Neutrophils	J. Phagocytosis

Human Blood Cells

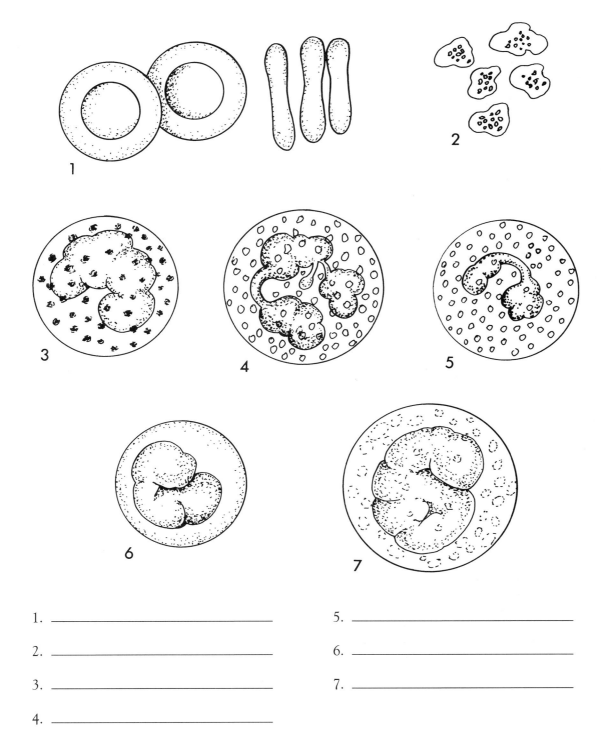

1. _____
2. _____
3. _____
4. _____

5. _____
6. _____
7. _____

Blood Typing

Using the key below, draw the appropriate reaction with the donor's blood in the circles.

Recipient's blood		Reactions with donor's blood			
RBC antigens	Plasma antibodies	Donor type O	Donor type A	Donor type B	Donor type AB
None (Type O)	Anti-A Anti-B	◯	◯	◯	◯
A (Type A)	Anti-B	◯	◯	◯	◯
B (Type B)	Anti-A	◯	◯	◯	◯
AB (Type AB)	(none)	◯	◯	◯	◯

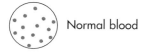 Normal blood   Agglutinated blood

CHAPTER 11

The Circulatory System

The heart is actually two pumps: one to move blood to the lungs, the other to push it out into the body. These two functions seem rather elementary by comparison to the complex and numerous functions performed by most of the other body organs, and yet, if either of these pumps stop, within a few short minutes all life ceases.

The heart is divided into two upper compartments, called atria or receiving chambers, and two lower compartments, called ventricles or discharging chambers. By the time a person reaches age 45, approximately 300,000 tons of blood will have passed through these chambers to be circulated to the blood vessels. These vessels—arteries, veins, and capillaries—serve different functions. Arteries carry blood from the heart, veins carry blood to the heart, and capillaries are exchange vessels or connecting links between the arteries and the veins. This closed system of circulation provides distribution of blood to the whole body (systemic circulation) and to specific regions, such as pulmonary circulation or hepatic portal circulation.

Blood pressure is the force of blood in the vessels. This force is highest in arteries and lowest in veins. Normal blood pressure varies among individuals and depends on the volume of blood in the arteries. The larger the volume of blood in the arteries, the more pressure is exerted on the walls of the arteries, and the higher the arterial pressure. Conversely, the less blood in the arteries, the lower the blood pressure.

A functional cardiovascular system is vital for survival because, without circulation, tissues would lack a supply of oxygen and nutrients. Waste products would begin to accumulate and could become toxic. Your review of this system will provide you with an understanding of the complex transportation mechanism of the body that is necessary for survival.

TOPICS FOR REVIEW

Before progressing to Chapter 12, you should have an understanding of the structure and function of the heart and the blood vessels. Your review should include a study of systemic, pulmonary, hepatic portal, and fetal circulations, and it should conclude with a thorough understanding of blood pressure and pulse.

HEART

Fill in the blanks.

1. Rhythmic compression of the heart combined with effective artificial respiration is known as _____.

2. The _____ _____ divides the heart into right and left sides between the atria.

3. The _____ are the two upper chambers of the heart.

4. The _____ are the two lower chambers of the heart.

5. The cardiac muscle tissue is referred to as the _____.

6. Inflammation of the heart lining is _____.

7. The two AV valves are _____ and _____.

8. _____ _____ involves the movement of blood from the right ventricle to the lungs.

9. An occlusion of a coronary artery is known as a _____ _____.

10. _____ _____ occurs when heart muscle cells are deprived of oxygen and become damaged or die.

11. The pacemaker of the heart is the _____ node.

12. A normal ECG tracing has three characteristic waves. They are _____, _____ _____, and _____ waves.

13. _____ begins just before the relaxation phase of cardiac muscle activity noted on an ECG.

Choose the correct term and write the letter in the space next to the appropriate definition below.

A. Pericardium
B. Severe chest pain
C. Thrombosis
D. Pulmonary
E. Heart block
F. Ventricles
G. Systemic

H. Coronary arteries
I. Systole
J. Depolarization
K. Atria
L. Apex
M. Epicardium

_____ 14. Covering of heart
_____ 15. Receiving chambers
_____ 16. Circulation from left ventricle throughout body
_____ 17. Blood clot
_____ 18. Semilunar valve
_____ 19. Discharging chambers
_____ 20. Supplies oxygen to heart muscle
_____ 21. Angina pectoris
_____ 22. Slow heart rate caused by blocked impulses
_____ 23. Contraction of the heart
_____ 24. Electrical activity associated with ECG
_____ 25. Blunt-pointed lower edge of heart
_____ 26. Visceral pericardium

If you have had difficulty with this section, review pages 274-283.

BLOOD VESSELS CIRCULATION

Match the term on the left with the proper selection on the right.

_____ 27. Arteries

_____ 28. Veins

_____ 29. Capillaries

_____ 30. Tunica adventitia

_____ 31. Precapillary sphincters

_____ 32. Superior vena cava

_____ 33. Aorta

A. Smooth muscle cells that guard entrance to capillaries

B. Carry blood to the heart

C. Carry blood into venules

D. Carry blood away from the heart

E. Largest vein

F. Largest artery

G. Outermost layer of arteries and veins

Circle the correct answer.

34. The aorta carries blood out of the:
    A. Right atrium
    B. Left atrium
    C. Right ventricle
    D. Left ventricle
    E. None of the above

35. The superior vena cava returns blood to the:
    A. Left atrium
    B. Left ventricle
    C. Right atrium
    D. Right ventricle
    E. None of the above

36. Which one of the following vessels has its wall made up entirely of endothelial cells?
    A. Vein
    B. Capillary
    C. Artery
    D. Venule
    E. Arteriole

37. The _____ is made up of smooth muscle.
    A. Tunica media
    B. Tunica adventitia
    C. Tunica intima
    D. Endothelium
    E. Myocardium

38. The _____ function as exchange vessels.
    A. Venules
    B. Capillaries
    C. Arteries
    D. Arterioles
    E. Veins

39. Blood returns from the lungs during pulmonary circulation via the:
    A. Pulmonary artery
    B. Pulmonary veins
    C. Aorta
    D. Inferior vena cava

40. The hepatic portal circulation serves the body by:
    A. Removing excess glucose and storing it in the liver as glycogen
    B. Detoxifying blood
    C. Removing various poisonous substances present in blood
    D. All of the above

41. The structure used to bypass the liver in fetal circulation is the:
    A. Foramen ovale
    B. Ductus venosus
    C. Ductus arteriosus
    D. Umbilical vein

42. The foramen ovale serves the fetal circulation by:
    A. Connecting the aorta and the pulmonary artery
    B. Shunting blood from the right atrium directly into the left atrium
    C. Bypassing the liver
    D. Bypassing the lungs

43. The structure used to connect the aorta and pulmonary artery in fetal circulation is the:
    A. Ductus arteriosus
    B. Ductus venosus
    C. Aorta
    D. Foramen ovale

44. Which of the following is *not* an artery?
    A. Femoral
    B. Popliteal
    C. Coronary
    D. Inferior vena cava

45. Which of the following has valves to assist the blood flow?
    A. Veins
    B. Arteries
    C. Capillaries
    D. Arterioles

 If you have had difficulty with this section, review pages 285-293.

BLOOD PRESSURE
PULSE

If the statement is true, write "T" in the answer blank. If the statement is false, correct the statement by circling the incorrect term and writing the correct term in the answer blank.

_____ 46. Blood pressure is highest in the veins and lowest in the arteries.

_____ 47. The difference between two blood pressures is referred to as blood pressure deficit.

_____ 48. If the blood pressure in the arteries were to decrease so that it became equal to the average pressure in the arterioles, circulation would increase.

_____ 49. A stroke is often the result of low blood pressure.

_____ 50. Massive hemorrhage increases blood pressure.

_____ 51. Blood pressure is the volume of blood in the vessels.

_____ 52. Both the strength and the rate of heartbeat affect cardiac output and blood pressure.

_____ 53. The diameter of the arterioles helps to determine how much blood drains out of arteries into arterioles.

_____ 54. A stronger heartbeat tends to decrease blood pressure and a weaker heartbeat tends to increase it.

_____ 55. The systolic pressure is the pressure while the ventricles relax.

_____ 56. The diastolic pressure is the pressure while the ventricles contract.

_____ 57. The pulse is a vein expanding and then recoiling.

_____ 58. The radial artery is located at the wrist.

_____ 59. The common carotid artery is located in the neck along the front edge of the sternocleidomastoid muscle.

_____ 60. The artery located at the bend of the elbow and used for locating the pulse is the dorsalis pedis.

 If you have had difficulty with this section, review pages 295-298.

UNSCRAMBLE THE WORDS

61. STMESYCI

62. NULVEE

63. RYTREA

64. USLEP

Take the circled letters, unscramble them, and fill in the statement.
How Noah survived the flood.

65. ☐☐☐☐☐☐

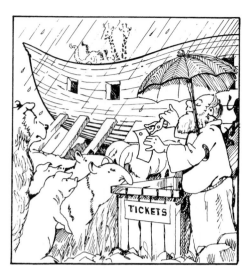

APPLYING WHAT YOU KNOW

66. Mr. Kehoe was experiencing angina pectoris. His doctor suggested a surgical procedure that would require the removal of a vein from another region of his body. This vein would then be used to bypass a partial blockage in his coronary arteries. What is this procedure called?

_____

67. Mr. Stuckey has heart block. His electrical impulses are being blocked from reaching the ventricles. An electrical device that causes ventricular contractions at a rate necessary to maintain circulation is being considered as possible treatment for his condition. What is this device called?

_____

68. Mrs. Heygood was diagnosed with an acute case of endocarditis. What is the real danger of this diagnosis?

_____

_____

_____

69. Mr. Philbrick returned from surgery in stable condition. The nurse noted that each time she took Mr. Philbrick's pulse and blood pressure, the pulse became higher and the blood pressure lower than the last time. What might be the cause?

_____

_____

_____

70. WORD FIND

Can you find 15 terms from this chapter? Words may be spelled top to bottom, bottom to top, right to left, left to right, or diagonally.

```
Y  H  Y  S  I  S  O  B  M  O  R  H  T  A  R
L  A  C  I  L  I  B  M  U  O  A  Y  N  I  Y
E  E  S  Y  S  T  E  M  I  C  C  G  D  E  U
M  V  E  N  U  L  E  D  D  C  I  X  M  D  I
E  Y  M  U  I  R  T  A  R  N  L  E  C  G  Y
N  O  I  T  A  Z  I  R  A  L  O  P  E  D  N
U  D  L  A  T  R  O  P  C  I  T  A  P  E  H
S  I  U  K  M  U  E  T  O  E  S  L  U  P  U
R  P  N  F  Y  C  B  E  D  R  A  L  Z  P  J
D  S  A  H  T  I  T  V  N  L  I  I  B  D  W
Q  U  R  O  I  V  A  Q  E  O  D  A  K  R  K
K  C  R  M  P  G  A  I  G  N  D  D  Z  Y  J
Y  I  Y  R  I  N  E  A  F  Z  L  Q  S  P  X
S  R  M  I  C  C  Q  O  A  W  U  N  H  O  K
P  T  A  V  H  H  Z  L  H  I  J  J  X  K  Z
```

Angina pectoris	ECG	Systemic
Apex	Endocardium	Thrombosis
Atrium	Hepatic portal	Tricuspid
Depolarization	Pulse	Umbilical
Diastolic	Semilunar	Venule

DID YOU KNOW?

- Your heart pumps more than 5 quarts of blood every minute—that's 2000 gallons a day.
- Every pound of excess fat contains some 200 miles of additional capillaries.

CIRCULATORY SYSTEM

Fill in the crossword puzzle.

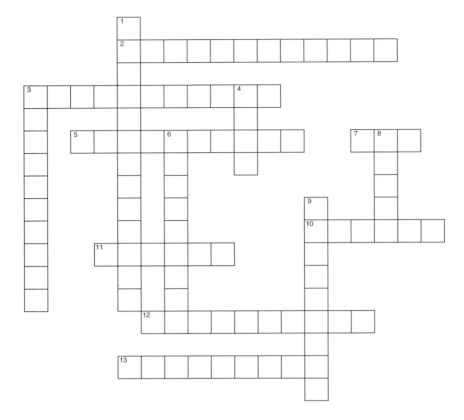

Across

2. Inflammation of the lining of the heart
3. Bicuspid valve (two words)
5. Inner layer of pericardium
7. Cardiopulmonary resuscitation (abbreviation)
10. Carries blood away from the heart
11. Upper chamber of the heart
12. Lower chambers of the heart
13. SA node

Down

1. Unique blood circulation through the liver (two words)
3. Muscular layer of the heart
4. Carries blood to the heart
6. Tiny artery
8. Heart rate
9. Carries blood from arterioles into venules

CHECK YOUR KNOWLEDGE

Multiple Choice

Circle the correct answer.

1. Systemic circulation involves movement of blood from the:
   A. Left ventricle throughout the body
   B. Right ventricle to the lungs
   C. Capillaries in visceral abdominal organs to the liver
   D. None of the above
2. What is the outside covering that surrounds and protects the heart called?
   A. Endocardium
   B. Myocardium
   C. Pericardium
   D. Ectocardium
3. What are the two upper heart chambers that receive blood from veins called?
   A. Chordae tendineae
   B. Atria
   C. Pericardia
   D. Ventricles
4. Which of the following events, if any, would *not* cause blood pressure to increase?
   A. Hemorrhaging
   B. Increasing the viscosity of blood
   C. Increasing the strength of the heartbeat
   D. All of the above events would cause blood pressure to increase
5. What are the components of the cardiovascular system that carry blood away from the heart called?
   A. Arteries
   B. Sinuses
   C. Veins
   D. Capillaries
6. Which of the following events, if any, does *not* precede contraction?
   A. P wave
   B. Atrial depolarization
   C. Ventricular depolarization
   D. All of these events precede contraction.
7. A structure called the foramen ovale connects which of the following?
   A. Right atrium and right ventricle
   B. Left atrium and left ventricle
   C. Right and left atria
   D. Right and left ventricles

8. What is the valve that permits blood to flow from the right ventricle into the pulmonary artery called?
    A. Tricuspid
    B. Mitral
    C. Aortic semilunar
    D. Pulmonary semilunar
9. To where does the superior vena cava carry blood?
    A. Left ventricle
    B. Coronary arteries
    C. Right atrium
    D. Pulmonary veins
10. What is the innermost coat of an artery that comes into direct contact with blood called?
    A. Lumen
    B. Tunica externa
    C. Tunica interna
    D. Turnica media

Matching

Select the most appropriate answer from column B for each item in column A. There is only one correct answer for each item.

Column A
_____ 11. Heart attack
_____ 12. QRS complex
_____ 13. Systole
_____ 14. Pulmonary circulation
_____ 15. Bicuspid
_____ 16. Hepatic portal circulation
_____ 17. Heart muscle
_____ 18. Pacemaker
_____ 19. T wave
_____ 20. Chest pain

Column B
A. Sinoatrial node
B. Liver
C. Myocardium
D. Ventricular repolarization
E. Angina pectoris
F. Myocardial infarction
G. Ventricular depolarization
H. Ventricular contraction
I. Lungs
J. Mitral

The Heart

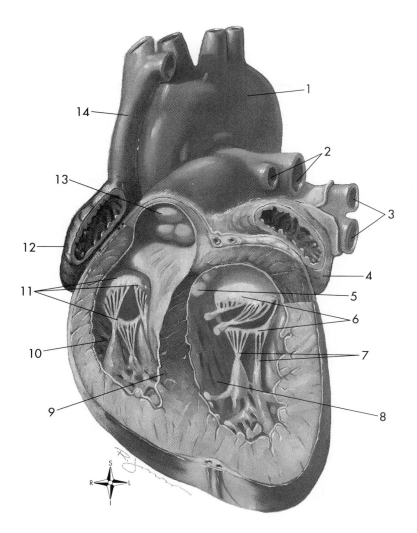

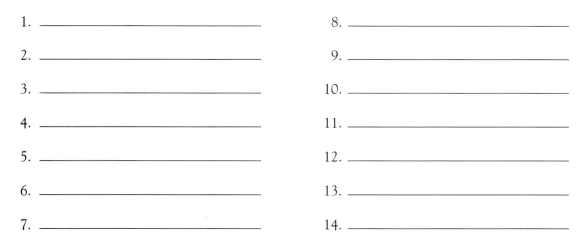

1. _____	8. _____
2. _____	9. _____
3. _____	10. _____
4. _____	11. _____
5. _____	12. _____
6. _____	13. _____
7. _____	14. _____

Conduction System of the Heart

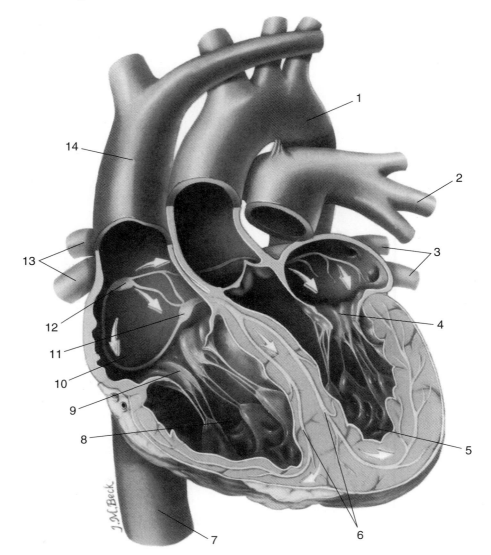

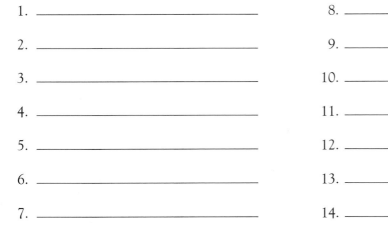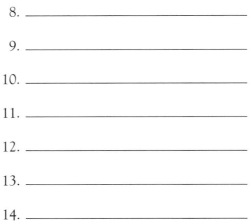

1. _____   8. _____

2. _____   9. _____

3. _____   10. _____

4. _____   11. _____

5. _____   12. _____

6. _____   13. _____

7. _____   14. _____

Fetal Circulation

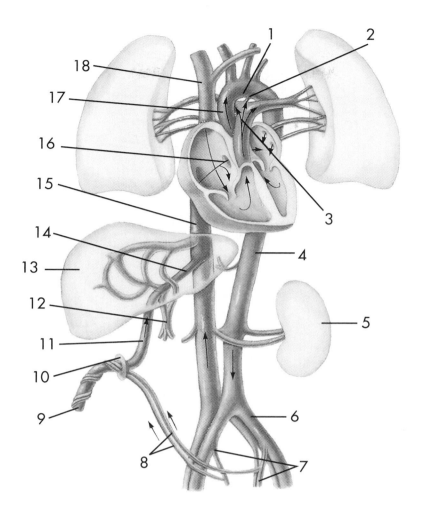

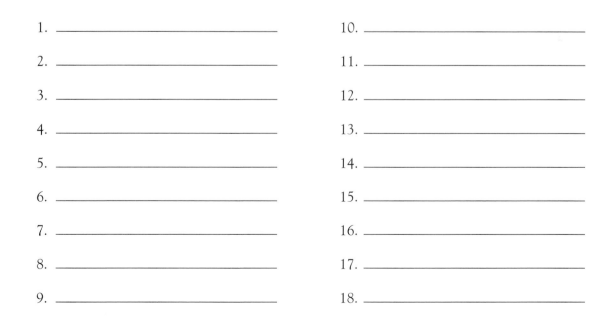

1. _____

2. _____

3. _____

4. _____

5. _____

6. _____

7. _____

8. _____

9. _____

10. _____

11. _____

12. _____

13. _____

14. _____

15. _____

16. _____

17. _____

18. _____

Hepatic Portal Circulation

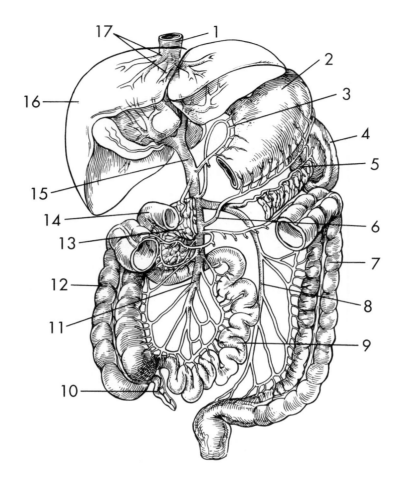

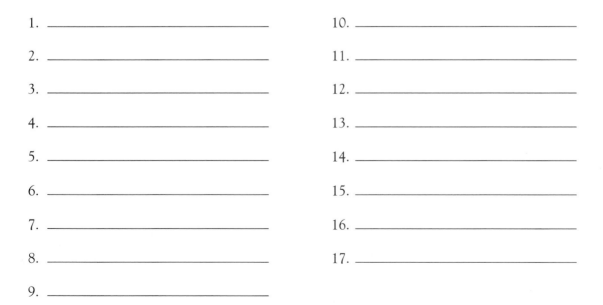

1. _____

2. _____

3. _____

4. _____

5. _____

6. _____

7. _____

8. _____

9. _____

10. _____

11. _____

12. _____

13. _____

14. _____

15. _____

16. _____

17. _____

Principal Arteries of the Body

1. _____
2. _____
3. _____
4. _____
5. _____
6. _____
7. _____
8. _____
9. _____
10. _____
11. _____
12. _____
13. _____
14. _____
15. _____
16. _____
17. _____
18. _____
19. _____
20. _____
21. _____
22. _____
23. _____
24. _____
25. _____
26. _____
27. _____
28. _____
29. _____
30. _____

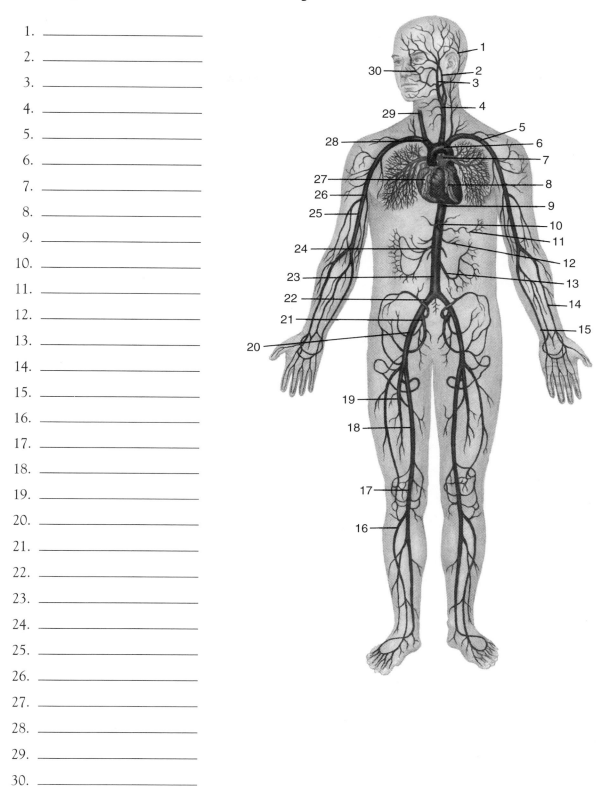

Principle Veins of the Body

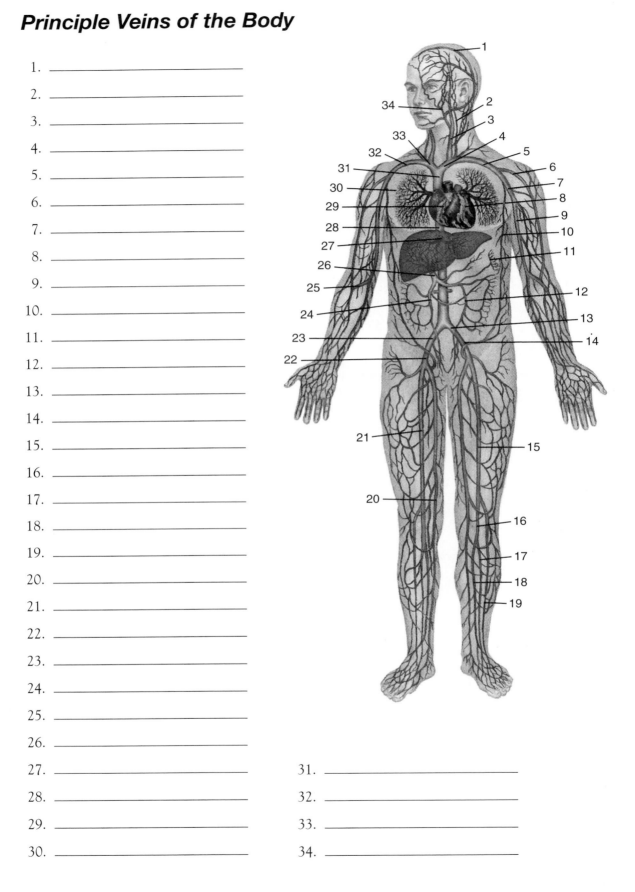

1. _____

2. _____

3. _____

4. _____

5. _____

6. _____

7. _____

8. _____

9. _____

10. _____

11. _____

12. _____

13. _____

14. _____

15. _____

16. _____

17. _____

18. _____

19. _____

20. _____

21. _____

22. _____

23. _____

24. _____

25. _____

26. _____

27. _____

28. _____

29. _____

30. _____

31. _____

32. _____

33. _____

34. _____

Normal ECG Deflections

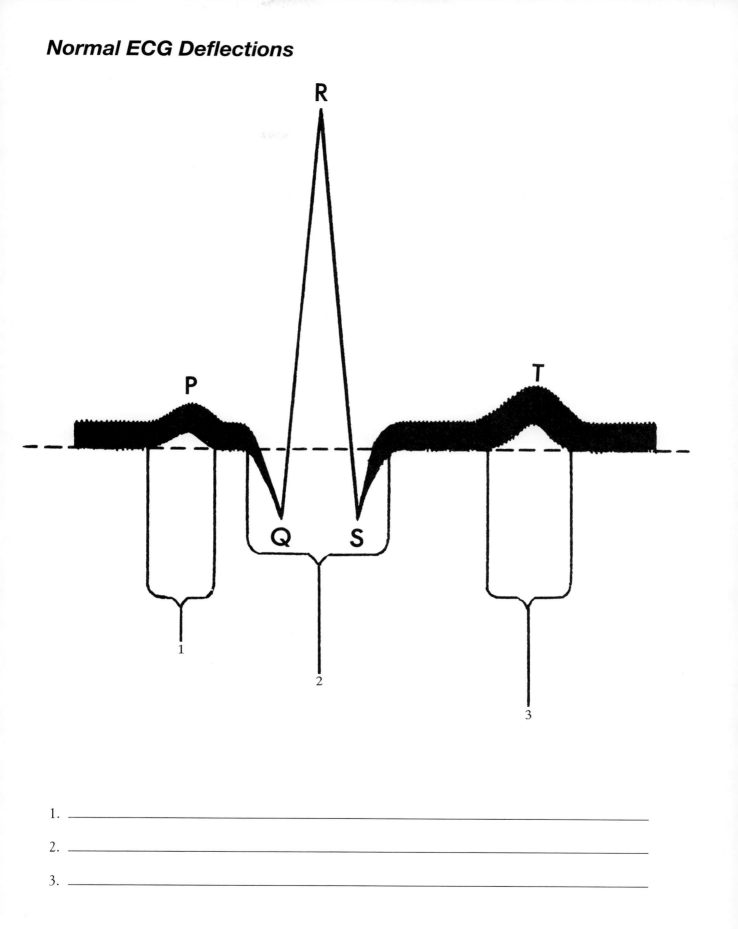

1. _____

2. _____

3. _____

CHAPTER 12

The Lymphatic System and Immunity

The lymphatic system is a system similar to the circulatory system. Lymph, like blood, flows through an elaborate route of vessels. In addition to lymphatic vessels, the lymphatic system consists of lymph nodes, lymph, and the spleen. Unlike the circulatory system, the lymphatic vessels do not form a closed circuit. Lymph flows only once through the vessels before draining into the general blood circulation. This system is a filtering mechanism for microorganisms and serves as a protective device against foreign invaders, such as cancer.

The immune system is the armed forces division of the body. Ready to attack at a moment's notice, the immune system defends us against the major enemies of the body: microorganisms, foreign transplanted tissue cells, and our own cells that have turned malignant.

The most numerous cells of the immune system are the lymphocytes. These cells circulate in the body's fluids seeking invading organisms and destroying them with powerful lymphotoxins, lymphokines, or antibodies.

Phagocytes, another large group of immune system cells, assist with the destruction of foreign invaders by a process known as phagocytosis. Neutrophils, monocytes, and connective tissue cells called macrophages use this process to surround unwanted microorganisms, ingest and digest them, and render them harmless to the body.

Another weapon that the immune system possesses is complement. Normally a group of inactive enzymes present in the blood, complement can be activated to kill invading cells by drilling holes in their cytoplasmic membranes, allowing fluid to enter the cell until it bursts.

Your review of this chapter will give you an understanding of how the body defends itself from the daily invasion of destructive substances.

TOPICS FOR REVIEW

Before progressing to Chapter 13, you should familiarize yourself with the functions of the lymphatic system, the immune system, and the major structures that make up these systems. Your review should include knowledge of lymphatic vessels, lymph nodes, lymph, antibodies, complement, and the development of B and T cells. Your study should conclude with an understanding of the differences in humoral and cell-mediated immunity.

THE LYMPHATIC SYSTEM

Fill in the blanks.

1. _____ is a specialized fluid formed in the tissue spaces that will be transported by way of specialized vessels to eventually reenter the circulatory system.

2. Blood plasma that has filtered out of capillaries into microscopic spaces between cells is called _____ _____.

3. The network of tiny blind-ended tubes distributed in the tissue spaces is called _____ _____.

4. Lymph eventually empties into two terminal vessels called the _____ _____ _____ and the _____ _____.

5. The thoracic duct has an enlarged pouch-like structure called the _____ _____.

6. Lymph is filtered by moving through _____ _____, which are located in clusters along the pathway of lymphatic vessels.

7. Lymph enters the node through four _____ lymph vessels.

8. Lymph exits from the node through a single _____ lymph vessel.

▶ *If you have had difficulty with this section, review pages 308-310.*

THYMUS
TONSILS
SPLEEN

Select the correct term from the options given and write the letter in the answer blank.

    A. Thymus   B. Tonsils   C. Spleen

_____ 9. Examples are palatine, pharyngeal, and lingual
_____ 10. Largest lymphoid organ in the body
_____ 11. Destroys worn out red blood cells
_____ 12. Located in the mediastinum
_____ 13. Serves as a reservoir for blood
_____ 14. T-lymphocytes
_____ 15. Largest at puberty

▶ *If you have had difficulty with this section, review page 311-312.*

THE IMMUNE SYSTEM

Match the term on the left with the proper selection on the right.

_____ 16. Nonspecific immunity   A. Inborn immunity
_____ 17. Inherited immunity   B. Natural immunity
_____ 18. Specific immunity   C. General protection
_____ 19. Acquired immunity   D. Artificial exposure
_____ 20. Immunization   E. Memory

IMMUNE SYSTEM MOLECULES

Choose the term that applies to each of the following descriptions. Write the letter for the term in the appropriate answer blank.

A. Antibodies
B. Antigen
C. Allergy
D. Anaphylactic shock
E. Monoclonal

F. Complement fixation
G. Complement
H. Humoral immunity
I. Combining site
J. hCG

_____ 21. Hypersensitivity of the immune system to harmless antigens
_____ 22. Life-threatening allergic reaction
_____ 23. Type of very specific antibodies produced from a population of identical cells
_____ 24. Protein compounds normally present in the body
_____ 25. Also known as antibody-mediated immunity
_____ 26. Combines with antibody to produce humoral immunity
_____ 27. Antibody
_____ 28. Process of changing molecule shape slightly to expose binding sites
_____ 29. Pregnancy test kits
_____ 30. Inactive proteins in blood

Circle the one that does **not** *belong.*

31. Antibody	Allergy	Protein compound	Combining site
32. Antigen	Invading cells	Foreign protein	Complement
33. Monoclonal	Antibodies	Antigen	Specific
34. Allergy	Complement	Anaphylactic shock	Antigen
35. Monoclonal	14	Complement	Proteins

 If you have had difficulty with this section, review pages 311-316.

IMMUNE SYSTEM CELLS

Circle the correct answer.

36. The most numerous cells of the immune system are the:
    A. Monocytes
    B. Eosinophils
    C. Neutrophils
    D. Lymphocytes
    E. Complement

37. Which of the terms listed below occurs third in the immune process?
    A. Plasma cells
    B. Stem cells
    C. Antibodies
    D. Activated B cells
    E. Immature B cells

38. Which one of the terms listed below occurs last in the immune process?
    A. Plasma cells
    B. Stem cells
    C. Antibodies
    D. Activated B cells
    E. Immature B cells

39. Moderate exercise has been found to:
    A. Decrease white blood cells
    B. Increase white blood cells
    C. Decrease platelets
    D. Decrease red blood cells

40. Which one of the following is part of the cell membrane of B cells?
    A. Complement
    B. Antigens
    C. Antibodies
    D. Epitopes
    E. None of the above

41. Immature B cells have:
    A. Four types of defense mechanisms on their cell membrane
    B. Several kinds of defense mechanisms on their cell membrane
    C. One specific kind of defense mechanism on their cell membrane
    D. No defense mechanisms on their cell membrane

42. Development of an immature B cell depends on the B cell coming in contact with:
    A. Complement
    B. Antibodies
    C. Lymphotoxins
    D. Lymphokines
    E. Antigens

43. The kind of cell that produces large numbers of antibodies is the:
    A. B cell
    B. Stem cell
    C. T cell
    D. Memory cell
    E. Plasma cell

44. Just one of these short-lived cells that make antibodies can produce _____ of them per second.
    A. 20
    B. 200
    C. 2000
    D. 20,000

45. Which of the following statements is *not* true of memory cells?
    A. They produce large numbers of antibodies.
    B. They are found in lymph nodes.
    C. They develop into plasma cells.
    D. They can react with antigens.
    E. All of the above are true of memory cells

46. T cell development begins in the:
    A. Lymph nodes
    B. Liver
    C. Pancreas
    D. Spleen
    E. Thymus
47. Human immunodeficiency virus (HIV) has its most obvious effects in:
    A. B cells
    B. Stem cells
    C. Plasma cells
    D. T cells
48. Interferon:
    A. Is produced by T cells within hours after infection by a virus
    B. Decreases the severity of many virus-related diseases
    C. Shows promise as an anticancer agent
    D. Has been shown to be effective in treating breast cancer
    E. All of the above
49. B cells function indirectly to produce:
    A. Humoral immunity
    B. Cell-mediated immunity
    C. Lymphotoxins
    D. Lymphokines
50. T cells function to produce:
    A. Humoral immunity
    B. Cell-mediated immunity
    C. Antibodies
    D. Memory cells

Fill in the blanks.
51. The first stage of development for B cells is called the _____
    _____.
52. The second stage of B cell development changes an immature B cell into a/an
    _____ _____ _____.
53. _____ _____ secrete copious amounts of antibody into the
    blood—nearly 2000 antibody molecules for every second they live.
54. T cells are lymphocytes that have undergone their first stage of development in the
    _____ _____.
55. _____ blocks HIV's ability to reproduce within infected cells.
56. _____ is a disease caused by a retrovirus that enters the bloodstream and inte-
    grates into the DNA of T cell lymphocytes.
57. Like many viruses, such as the common cold, HIV changes rapidly so the development of a
    _____ may not occur for several years.

If you have had difficulty with this section, review pages 310-322.

UNSCRAMBLE THE WORDS

58. NTCMPEOLEM

59. MTMYIUNI

60. OENCLS

61. FNROERTENI

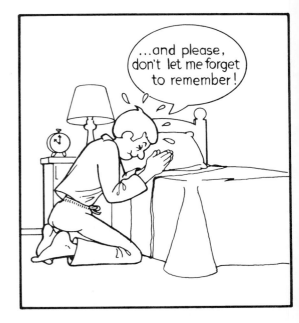

Take the circled letters, unscramble them, and fill in the statement.

What the student was praying for the night before exams.

APPLYING WHAT YOU KNOW

63. Two-year-old baby Metcalfe was exposed to chickenpox. He had been a particularly sickly child, and so the doctor decided to give him a dose of Interferon. What effect was the physician hoping for in baby Metcalfe's case?

_____

_____

64. Marcia was an intravenous drug user. She was recently diagnosed with Kaposi's sarcoma. What is another possible diagnosis?

_____

65. Baby Phelps was born without a thymus gland. Immediate plans were made for a transplant to be performed. In the meantime, baby Phelps was placed in strict isolation. Why was this done?

_____

_____

_____

156   Chapter 12: The Lymphatic System and Immunity

Can you find 14 terms from this chapter? Words may be spelled top to bottom, bottom to top, right to left, left to right, or diagonally.

```
I  N  F  L  A  M  M  A  T  O  R  Y  F  C  G
Q  N  L  O  Y  Z  O  C  C  P  A  O  F  S  X
M  W  T  A  A  M  N  J  X  Q  K  R  N  P  H
U  R  L  E  R  M  P  X  B  R  U  I  A  L  C
C  M  A  C  R  O  P  H  A  G  E  I  E  D  Z
X  M  N  D  K  F  M  N  O  T  U  C  R  N  M
A  E  O  R  E  Z  E  U  O  C  F  B  Y  E  B
Y  P  L  E  B  G  G  R  H  T  Y  T  S  E  D
Y  S  C  R  I  S  P  J  O  E  I  T  M  L  A
Z  M  O  T  J  X  E  T  O  N  A  E  E  P  X
T  O  N  S  I  L  S  S  U  M  Y  H  T  S  Y
W  A  O  C  J  N  I  M  W  K  O  Z  E  N  D
D  W  M  K  W  R  M  O  I  P  S  H  Y  B  G
F  H  W  U  J  I  Z  F  V  D  Z  L  Y  T  X
```

Acquired	Interferon	Proteins
Antigen	Lymph	Spleen
Humoral	Lymphocytes	Thymus
Immunity	Macrophage	Tonsils
Inflammatory	Monoclonal	

DID YOU KNOW?

In the United States, the HIV infection rate is increasing four times faster in women than in men. Women tend to underestimate their risk.

LYMPH AND IMMUNITY

Fill in the crossword puzzle.

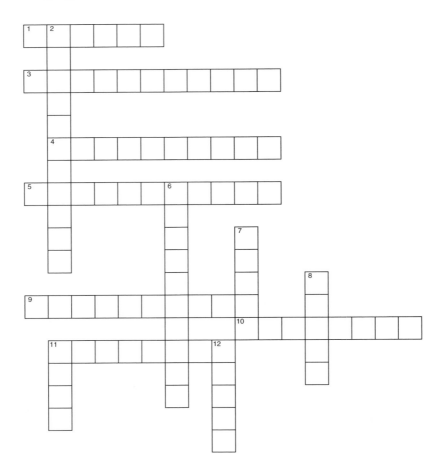

Across

1. Largest lymphoid organ in the body
3. Connective tissue cells that are phagocytes
4. Protein compounds normally present in the body
5. Remain in reserve then turn into plasma cells when needed (two words)
9. Synthetically produced to fight certain diseases
10. Lymph exits the node through this lymph vessel
11. Lymph enters the node through these lymph vessels

Down

2. Secretes a copious amount of antibodies into the blood (two words)
6. Inactive proteins
7. Family of identical cells descended from one cell
8. Type of lymphocyte (humoral immunity; two words)
11. Immune deficiency disorder
12. Type of lymphocyte (cell-mediated immunity; two words)

CHECK YOUR KNOWLEDGE

Multiple Choice

Circle the correct answer.

1. T cells do which of the following?
   A. Develop in the thymus.
   B. Form memory cells.
   C. Form plasma cells.
   D. All of the above

2. Lymph does which of the following?
   A. Forms as blood plasma filters out of capillaries.
   B. Empties into the heart.
   C. Flows through lymphatic arteries.
   D. All of the above

3. Acquired immune deficiency syndrome is characterized by which of the following?
   A. Caused by a retro virus.
   B. Causes inadequate T-cell formation.
   C. Can result in death caused by cancer or infection.
   D. All of the above

4. Interferon is:
   A. Produced by B cells
   B. A protein compound that protects other cells by interfering with the ability of a virus to reproduce
   C. A group of inactive enzyme proteins normally present in blood
   D. All of the above

5. B cells do which of the following?
   A. Develop into plasma cells and memory cells.
   B. Establish humoral immunity.
   C. Develop from primitive cells in bone marrow called stem cells.
   D. All of the above

6. Which of the following kills invading cells by drilling a hole in the plasma membrane?
   A. Interferon
   B. Complement
   C. Antibody
   D. Memory cell

7. Which of the following cell types functions in the immune system?
   A. Macrophages
   B. Lymphocytes
   C. T cells
   D. All of the above

8. Which of the following are phagocytes?
   A. Kupffer's cells
   B. Dust cells
   C. Macrophages
   D. All of the above
9. What is a rapidly growing population of identical cells that produce large quantities of specific antibodies called?
   A. Complementary
   B. Lymphotoxic
   C. Chemotactic
   D. Monoclonal
10. Which of the following is a form of passive natural immunity?
   A. A child develops measles and acquires an immunity to subsequent infection.
   B. Antibodies are injected into an infected individual.
   C. An infant receives protection through its mother's milk.
   D. Vaccinations are given against smallpox.

Matching

Select the most appropriate answer from column B for each item in column A. There is only one correct answer for each item.

Column A
_____ 11. Adenoids
_____ 12. B cell
_____ 13. Clone
_____ 14. HIV virus
_____ 15. Complement
_____ 16. Filtration
_____ 17. Cisterna chyli
_____ 18. T cell
_____ 19. Vaccination
_____ 20. Antigen

Column B
A. Thoracic duct
B. Lymph node
C. Artificial immunity
D. Humoral immunity
E. Pharyngeal tonsils
F. Foreign protein
G. Inactive enzymes
H. AIDS
I. Identical cells
J. Cell-mediated immunity

B Cell Development

Complete the diagram:

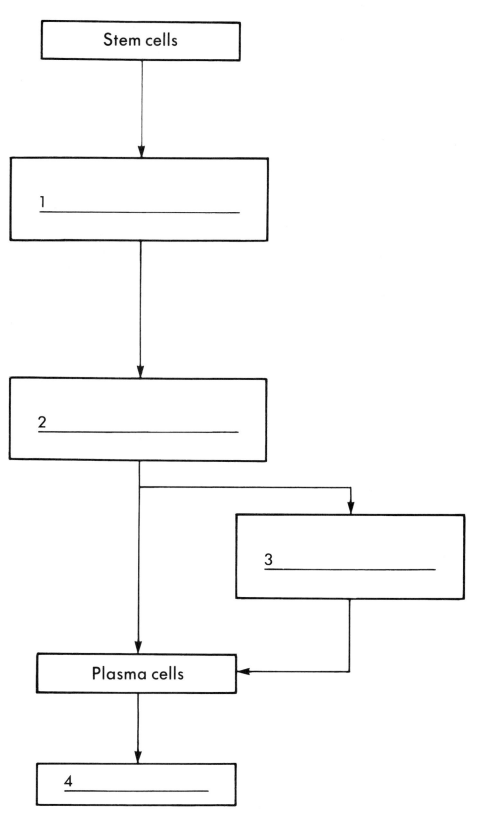

Function of Sensitized T Cells

Complete the diagram:

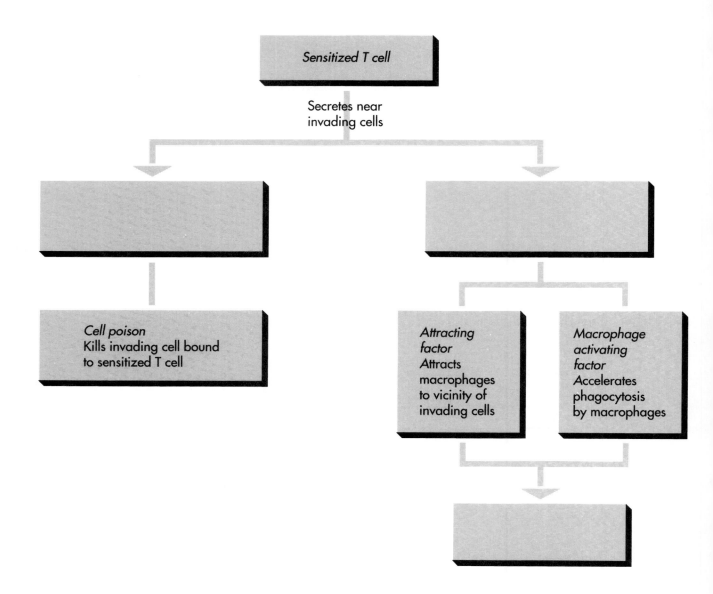

Sensitized T cell

Secretes near
invading cells

Cell poison
Kills invading cell bound
to sensitized T cell

Attracting
factor
Attracts
macrophages
to vicinity of
invading cells

Macrophage
activating
factor
Accelerates
phagocytosis
by macrophages

Principal Organs of the Lymphatic System

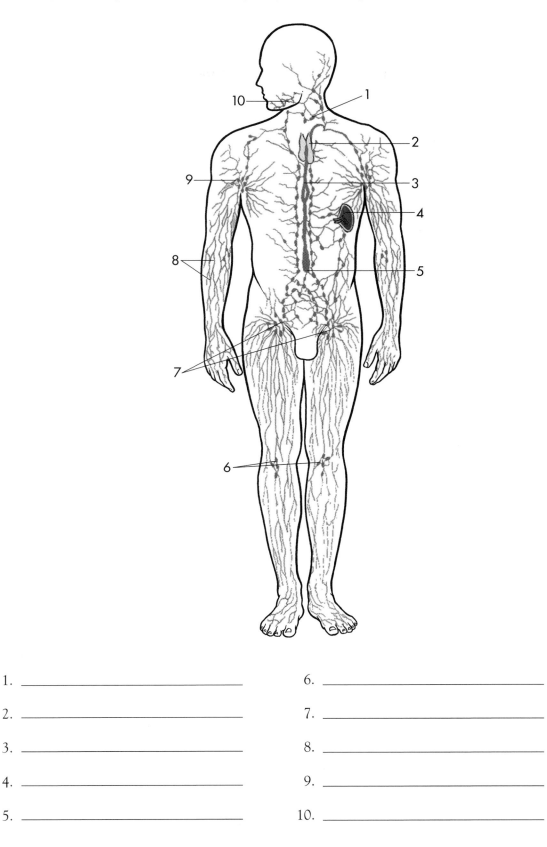

1. _____
2. _____
3. _____
4. _____
5. _____

6. _____
7. _____
8. _____
9. _____
10. _____

Chapter 12: The Lymphatic System and Immunity   163

CHAPTER 13 The Respiratory System

As you sit reviewing this system, your body needs 16 quarts of air per minute. Walking requires 24 quarts of air per minute, and running requires 50 quarts per minute. The respiratory system provides the air necessary for you to perform your daily activities and eliminates the waste gases from the air that you breathe. Take a deep breath, and think of the air entering some 250 million tiny air sacs that are similar in appearance to clusters of grapes. These microscopic air sacs expand to let air in and contract to force it out. These tiny sacs, alveoli, are the functioning units of the respiratory system. They provide the necessary volume of oxygen and eliminate carbon dioxide 24 hours a day.

Air enters either through the mouth or the nasal cavity. It next passes through the pharynx and past the epiglottis, then through the glottis and the rest of the larynx. It continues down the trachea, into the bronchi to the bronchioles, and finally through the alveoli. The reverse occurs for expelled air.

The exchange of gases between air in the lungs and in the blood is known as external respiration. The exchange of gases that occurs between the blood and the cells of the body is known as internal respiration. By constantly supplying adequate oxygen and by removing carbon dioxide as it forms, the respiratory system helps to maintain an environment conducive to maximum cell efficiency.

Your review of this system is necessary to provide you with an understanding of this essential homeostatic mechanism.

TOPICS FOR REVIEW

Before progressing to Chapter 14, you should have an understanding of the structure and function of the organs of the respiratory system. Your review should include knowledge of the mechanisms responsible for both internal and external respiration. Your study should conclude with a knowledge of the volumes of air exchanged in pulmonary ventilation and an understanding of how respiration is regulated.

STRUCTURAL PLAN
RESPIRATORY TRACTS
RESPIRATORY MUCOSA

Match the term with the definition.

A. Diffusion
B. Respiratory membrane
C. Alveoli
D. URI
E. Respiration

F. Respiratory mucosa
G. Upper respiratory tract
H. Lower respiratory tract
I. Cilia
J. Air distributor

_____ 1. Function of respiratory system
_____ 2. Pharynx
_____ 3. Passive transport process responsible for actual exchange of gases
_____ 4. Assists with the movement of mucus toward the pharynx
_____ 5. Barrier between the blood in the capillaries and the air in the alveolus
_____ 6. Lines the tubes of the respiratory tree
_____ 7. Terminal air sacs
_____ 8. Trachea
_____ 9. Head cold
_____ 10. Homeostatic mechanism

Fill in the blanks.

The organs of the respiratory system are designed to perform two basic functions. They serve as an:
(11) _____ _____ and as a (12) _____
_____. In addition to the above, the respiratory system (13) _____,
(14) _____, and (15) _____ the air we breathe. Respiratory
organs include the (16) _____, (17) _____, (18) _____,
(19) _____, (20) _____, and the (21) _____.
The respiratory system ends in millions of tiny, thin-walled sacs called (22) _____.
(23) _____ of gases takes place in these sacs. Two aspects of the structure of these
sacs assist them in the exchange of gases. First, an extremely thin membrane, the (24)
_____ _____, allows for easy exchange, and second, the large
number of air sacs makes an enormous (25) _____ area.

▶ *If you have had difficulty with this section, review pages 331-335.*

NOSE
PHARYNX
LARYNX

Circle the one that does not belong.

| 26. Nares | Septum | Oropharynx | Conchae |
| 27. Conchae | Frontal | Maxillary | Sphenoidal |

166   Chapter 13: Respiratory System

28. Oropharynx	Throat	5 inches	Epiglottis
29. Pharyngeal	Adenoids	Uvula	Nasopharynx
30. Middle ear	Tubes	Nasopharynx	Larynx
31. Voice box	Thyroid cartilage	Tonsils	Vocal cords
32. Palatine	Eustachian tube	Tonsils	Oropharynx
33. Pharynx	Epiglottis	Adam's apple	Voice box

Select the correct term from the options given and write the letter in the answer blank.

A. Nose   B. Pharynx   C. Larynx

_____ 34. Warms and humidifies air

_____ 35. Air and food pass through here

_____ 36. Sinuses

_____ 37. Conchae

_____ 38. Septum

_____ 39. Tonsils

_____ 40. Middle ear infections

_____ 41. Epiglottis

 If you have had difficulty with this section, review pages 335-338.

TRACHEA
BRONCHI, BRONCHIOLES, AND ALVEOLI
LUNGS AND PLEURA

Fill in the blanks.

42. The windpipe is more properly referred to as the _____.

43. _____ keeps the framework of the trachea almost noncollapsible.

44. A lifesaving technique designed to free the trachea of ingested food or foreign objects is the _____ _____.

45. The first branch or division of the trachea leading to the lungs is the _____ _____.

46. Each alveolar duct ends in several _____ _____.

47. The narrow part of each lung, up under the collarbone, is its _____.

48. The _____ covers the outer surface of the lungs and lines the inner surface of the rib cage.

49. Inflammation of the lining of the thoracic cavity is _____.

50. The presence of air in the pleural space on one side of the chest is a _____.

 If you have had difficulty with this section, review pages 338-344.

RESPIRATION

If the statement is true, write "T" in the answer blank. If the statement is false, correct the statement by circling the incorrect term and writing the correct term in the answer blank.

_____ 51. Diffusion is the process that moves air into and out of the lungs.

_____ 52. For inspiration to take place, the diaphragm and other respiratory muscles relax.

_____ 53. Diffusion is a passive process that results in movement up a concentration gradient.

_____ 54. The exchange of gases that occurs between blood in tissue capillaries and the body cells is external respiration.

_____ 55. Many pulmonary volumes can be measured as a person breathes into a spirometer.

_____ 56. Ordinarily we take about 2 pints of air into our lungs.

_____ 57. The amount of air normally breathed in and out with each breath is called tidal volume.

_____ 58. The largest amount of air that one can breathe out in one expiration is called residual volume.

_____ 59. The inspiratory reserve volume is the amount of air that can be forcibly inhaled after a normal inspiration.

▶ *If you have had difficulty with this section, review pages 346-349.*

Circle the best answer.

60. The term that means the same thing as breathing is:
    A. Gas exchange
    B. Respiration
    C. Inspiration
    D. Expiration
    E. Pulmonary ventilation

61. Carbaminohemoglobin is formed when _____ binds to hemoglobin.
    A. Oxygen
    B. Amino acids
    C. Carbon dioxide
    D. Nitrogen
    E. None of the above

62. Most of the oxygen transported by the blood is:
    A. Dissolved in white blood cells
    B. Bound to white blood cells
    C. Bound to hemoglobin
    D. Bound to carbaminohemoglobin
    E. None of the above

63. Which of the following would *not* assist inspiration?
    A. Elevation of the ribs
    B. Elevation of the diaphragm
    C. Contraction of the diaphragm
    D. Chest cavity becomes longer from top to bottom
64. A young adult male would have a vital capacity of about _____ mL.
    A. 500
    B. 1200
    C. 3300
    D. 4800
    E. 6200
65. The amount of air that can be forcibly exhaled after expiring the tidal volume is known as the:
    A. Total lung capacity
    B. Vital capacity
    C. Inspiratory reserve volume
    D. Expiratory reserve volume
    E. None of the above
66. Which one of the following is correct?
    A. VC = TV − IRV + ERV
    B. VC = TV + IRV − ERV
    C. VC = TV + IRV × ERV
    D. VC = TV + IRV + ERV
    E. None of the above

▷ *If you have had difficulty with this section, review pages 346-349.*

REGULATION OF RESPIRATION
RECEPTORS INFLUENCING RESPIRATION
TYPES OF BREATHING

Match the term on the left with the proper selection on the right.

_____ 67. Inspiratory center

_____ 68. Chemoreceptors

_____ 69. Pulmonary stretch receptors

_____ 70. Dyspnea

_____ 71. Respiratory arrest

_____ 72. Eupnea

_____ 73. Hypoventilation

A. Difficult breathing
B. Located in carotid bodies
C. Slow and shallow respirations
D. Normal respiratory rate
E. Located in the medulla
F. Failure to resume breathing following a period of apnea
G. Located throughout pulmonary airways and in the alveoli

▷ *If you have had difficulty with this section, review page 351.*

UNSCRAMBLE THE WORDS

74. SPUELIRY

75. CRNBOSITHI

76. SESXPTIAI

77. DDNEAOIS

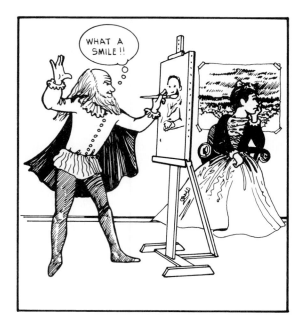

Take the circled letters, unscramble them, and fill in the statement.

What Mona Lisa was to DaVinci.

78.

APPLYING WHAT YOU KNOW

79. Mr. Gorski is a heavy smoker. Recently he has noticed that when he gets up in the morning he has a bothersome cough that brings up a large accumulation of mucus. This cough persists for several minutes and then leaves until the next morning. What is an explanation for this problem?

_____

_____

_____

_____

80. Kim was 5 years old and was a mouth breather. She had repeated episodes of tonsillitis, and her pediatrician suggested removal of her tonsils and adenoids. He further suggested that the surgery would probably cure her mouth-breathing problem. Why is this a possibility?

_____

_____

_____

_____

81. WORD FIND

Can you find 14 terms from this chapter? Words may be spelled top to bottom, bottom to top, right to left, left to right, or diagonally.

```
N  K  S  A  Q  B  I  L  V  A  D  T  I  X  D
O  X  O  O  B  F  I  F  G  I  M  N  R  G  Y
I  G  N  X  W  D  E  E  F  L  B  A  U  T  S
T  B  K  Y  N  H  E  F  O  I  U  T  I  R  P
A  T  M  H  E  O  U  T  R  C  C  C  P  V  N
L  L  A  E  P  S  I  R  I  Z  A  A  N  F  E
I  P  T  M  I  H  G  T  I  P  R  F  P  C  A
T  U  B  O  G  Q  E  V  A  Q  O  R  V  N  W
N  L  N  G  L  R  J  C  C  R  T  U  P  D  C
E  M  U  L  O  V  L  A  U  D  I  S  E  R  E
V  O  V  O  T  A  N  G  J  E  D  P  Z  U  U
O  N  K  B  T  C  N  U  U  E  B  O  S  J  S
P  A  L  I  I  K  E  U  C  N  O  Z  K  N  A
Y  R  V  N  S  D  I  O  N  E  D  A  M  F  I
H  Y  O  M  L  O  A  Z  D  T  Y  M  N  L  K
```

Adenoids   Epiglottis   Residual volume
Carotid body   Hypoventilation   Surfactant
Cilia   Inspiration   URI
Diffusion   Oxyhemoglobin   Vital capacity
Dyspnea   Pulmonary

DID YOU KNOW?

If the alveoli in our lungs were flattened out, they would cover a half of a tennis court.

RESPIRATORY SYSTEM

Fill in the crossword puzzle.

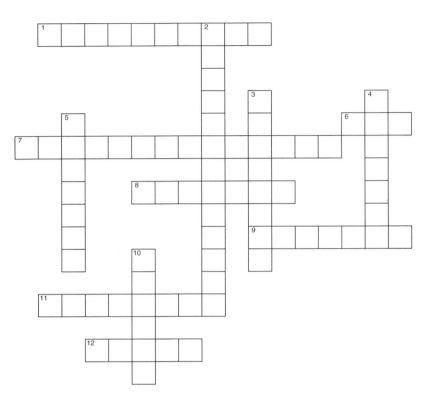

Across

1. Device used to measure the amount of air exchanged in breathing
6. Expiratory reserve volume (abbreviation)
7. Sphenoidal (two words)
8. Terminal air sacs
9. Shelf-like structures that protrude into the nasal cavity
11. Inflammation of pleura
12. Respirations stop

Down

2. Surgical procedure to remove tonsils
3. Doctor who developed lifesaving technique
4. Windpipe
5. Trachea branches into right and left structures
10. Voice box

CHECK YOUR KNOWLEDGE

Multiple Choice

Circle the correct answer.

1. Chemoreceptors in the carotid and aortic bodies are characterized by which of the following?
   A. Sensitive to increases in blood carbon dioxide level
   B. Found in the brain
   C. Sensitive to increases in blood oxygen level
   D. Send impulses to the heart

2. What is the lowest segment of the pharynx called?
   A. Oropharynx
   B. Laryngopharynx
   C. Nasopharynx
   D. Hypopharynx

3. What is the narrow upper portion of a lung called?
   A. Base
   B. Notch
   C. Costal surface
   D. Apex

4. What is the largest amount of air that we can breathe in and out in one inspiration and expiration called?
   A. Tidal volume
   B. Vital capacity
   C. Residual volume
   D. Inspiratory reserve volume

5. Which of the following statements, if any, does *not* describe a characteristic of human lungs?
   A. Both right and left lungs are composed of three lobes.
   B. Bronchi subdivide to form bronchioles.
   C. Capillary supply is abundant to facilitate gas exchange.
   D. All of the above statements are characteristic of human lungs

6. Which body function is made possible by the existence of fibrous bands stretched across the larynx?
   A. Swallowing
   B. Breathing
   C. Diffusion
   D. Speech

7. The trachea is made almost noncollapsible by the presence of which of the following?
   A. Rings of cartilage
   B. Thyroid cartilage
   C. Epiglottis
   D. Vocal cords

8. Which of the following is *true* of the exchange of respiratory gases between the lungs and the blood?
   A. It takes place by diffusion.
   B. It is called external respiration.
   C. Both A and B are true
   D. None of the above is true
9. When the diaphragm contracts, which phase of ventilation is taking place?
   A. External respiration
   B. Expiration
   C. Internal respiration
   D. Inspiration
10. Which of the following is *not* characteristic of the nasal cavities?
    A. They contain many blood vessels that warm incoming air.
    B. They contain the adenoids.
    C. They are lined with mucous membranes.
    D. They are separated by a partition called the nasal septum.

Matching

Select the most appropriate answer from column B for each item in column A. There is only one correct answer for each item.

Column A	Column B
_____ 11. Vocal cords	A. Serous membrane
_____ 12. Pulmonary ventilation	B. Pharynx
_____ 13. Pleura	C. Paranasal sinus
_____ 14. Pneumothorax	D. LVRS
_____ 15. Emphysema	E. Larynx
_____ 16. Throat	F. Diffusion
_____ 17. Ethmoidal	G. Collapsed lung
_____ 18. Windpipe	H. Trachea
_____ 19. Alveoli	I. Breathing
_____ 20. Surfactant	J. IRDS

Sagittal View of Face and Neck

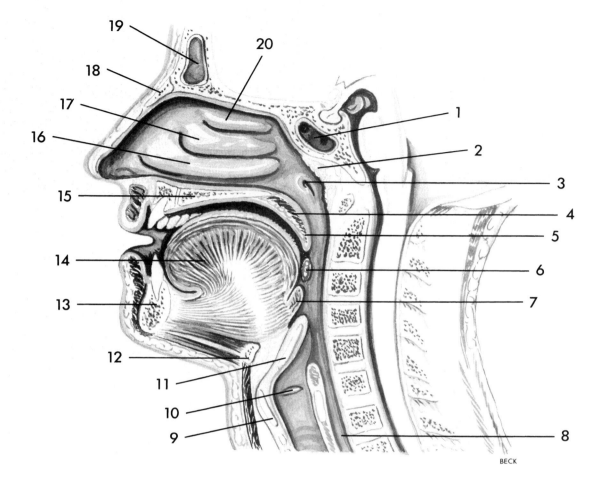

BECK

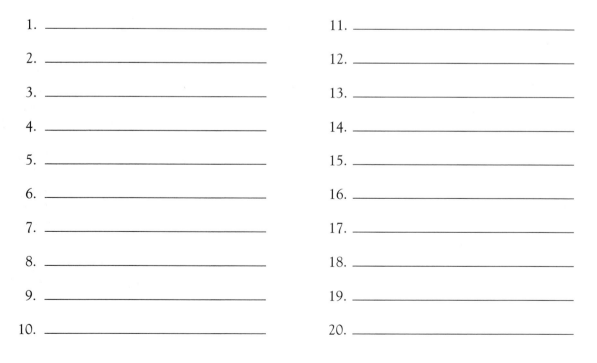

Respiratory Organs

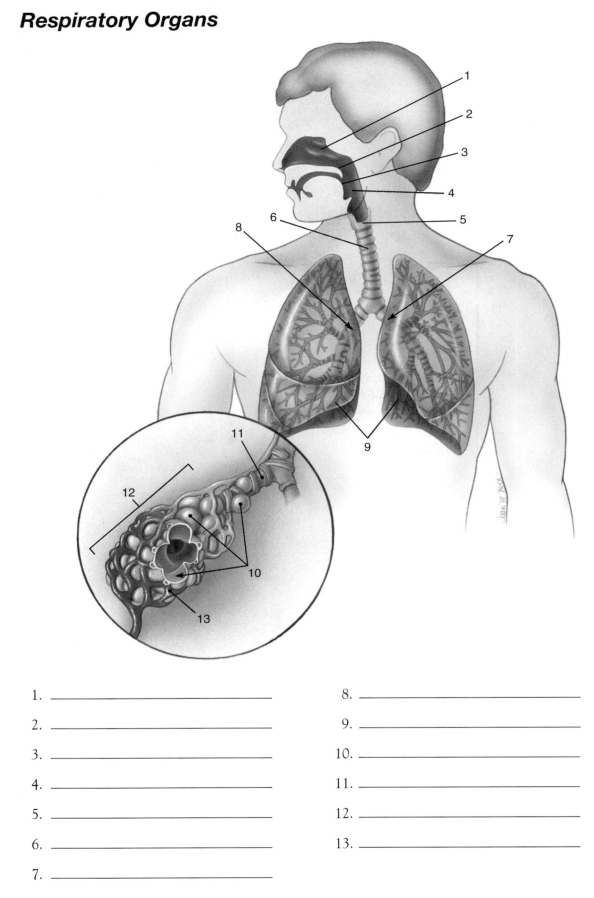

1. _____

2. _____

3. _____

4. _____

5. _____

6. _____

7. _____

8. _____

9. _____

10. _____

11. _____

12. _____

13. _____

Pulmonary Ventilation Volumes

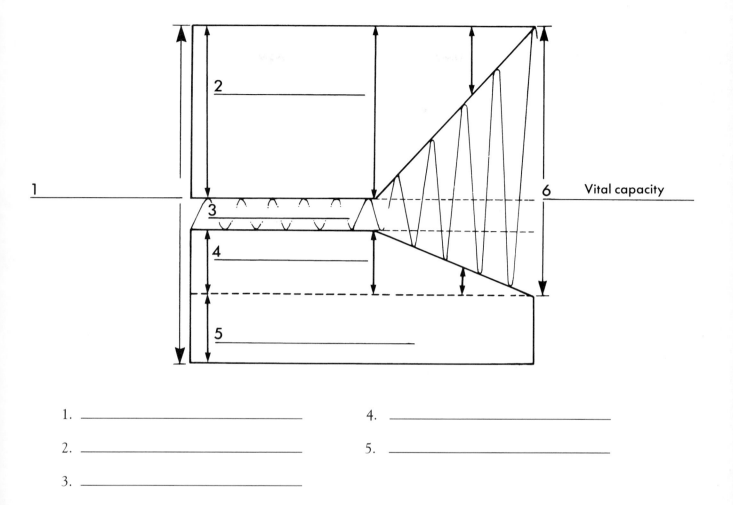

1. _____   4. _____

2. _____   5. _____

3. _____

CHAPTER **14** # The Digestive System

Think of the last meal you ate. Imagine the different shapes, sizes, tastes, and textures that you so recently enjoyed. Think of those items circulating in your bloodstream in those same original shapes and sizes. Impossible? Of course. And because of this impossibility, you will begin to understand and marvel at the close relationship of the digestive system to the circulatory system. It is the digestive system that changes our food, both mechanically and chemically, into a form that is acceptable to both the blood and the body.

This change begins the moment you take the very first bite. Digestion starts in the mouth, where food is chewed and mixed with saliva. The food then moves down the pharynx and esophagus by peristalsis and enters the stomach. In the stomach it is churned and mixed with gastric juices to become chyme. The chyme goes from the stomach to the duodenum where it is further broken down chemically by intestinal fluids, bile, and pancreatic juice. Those secretions prepare the food for absorption all along the course of the small intestine.

Products that are not absorbed pass on through the entire length of the small intestine (duodenum, jejunum, ileum). From there they enter into the cecum of the large intestine, then the ascending colon, transverse colon, descending colon, sigmoid colon, into the rectum and out the anus.

Products that are used in the cells undergo absorption. Absorption allows newly processed nutrients to pass through the walls of the digestive tract and into the bloodstream to be distributed to the cells.

Your review of this system will help you understand the mechanical and chemical processes necessary to convert food into energy sources and compounds necessary for survival.

TOPICS FOR REVIEW

Before progressing to Chapter 15, you should review the structure and function of all the organs of digestion. You should have an understanding of the process of digestion, both chemical and mechanical, and of the processes of absorption and metabolism.

WALL OF THE DIGESTIVE SYSTEM

Fill in the blanks.

1. The organs of the digestive system form an irregularly shaped tube called the alimentary canal or the _____ _____.
2. The churning of food in the stomach is an example of the _____ breakdown of food.
3. _____ breakdown occurs when digestive enzymes act on food as it passes through the digestive tract.
4. Waste material resulting from the digestive process is known as _____.
5. Foods undergo three kinds of processing in the body: _____, _____, and _____.
6. The serosa of the digestive tube is composed of the _____ _____ in the abdominal cavity.
7. The digestive tract extends from the _____ to the _____.
8. The inside or hollow space within the alimentary canal is called the _____.
9. The inside layer of the digestive tract is the _____.
10. The connective tissue layer that lies beneath the lining of the digestive tract is the _____.
11. The muscularis contracts and moves food through the gastrointestinal tract by a process known as _____.
12. The outermost covering of the digestive tube is the _____.
13. The loops of the digestive tract are anchored to the posterior wall of the abdominal cavity by the _____.

Select the correct term from the choices given and write the letter in the answer blank.

       A. Main organ   B. Accessory organ

_____ 14. Mouth
_____ 15. Parotids
_____ 16. Liver
_____ 17. Stomach
_____ 18. Cecum
_____ 19. Esophagus
_____ 20. Rectum
_____ 21. Pharynx
_____ 22. Appendix
_____ 23. Teeth
_____ 24. Gallbladder
_____ 25. Pancreas

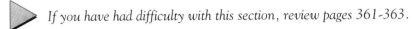 *If you have had difficulty with this section, review pages 361-363.*

MOUTH
TEETH
SALIVARY GLANDS

Circle the best answer.

26. Which one of the following is *not* a part of the roof of the mouth?
    A. Uvula
    B. Palatine bones
    C. Maxillary bones
    D. Soft palate
    E. All of the above are part of the roof of the mouth

27. The largest of the papillae on the surface of the tongue are the:
    A. Filiform
    B. Fungiform
    C. Vallate
    D. Taste buds

28. The first baby tooth, on an average, appears at age:
    A. 2 months
    B. 1 year
    C. 3 months
    D. 1 month
    E. 6 months

29. The portion of the tooth that is covered with enamel is the:
    A. Pulp cavity
    B. Neck
    C. Root
    D. Crown
    E. None of the above

30. The wall of the pulp cavity is surrounded by:
    A. Enamel
    B. Dentin
    C. Cementum
    D. Connective tissue
    E. Blood and lymphatic vessels

31. Which of the following teeth is missing from the deciduous arch?
    A. Central incisor
    B. Canine
    C. Second premolar
    D. First molar
    E. Second molar

32. The permanent central incisor erupts between the ages of:
    A. 9-13
    B. 5-6
    C. 7-10
    D. 7-8
    E. None of the above

33. The third molar appears between the ages of:
    A. 10-14
    B. 5-8
    C. 11-16
    D. 17-24
    E. None of the above
34. Which one of the following will *not* significantly reduce caries?
    A. Reduction of plaque accumulation on teeth
    B. Fluoride in the water supply
    C. Regular and thorough brushing
    D. Eating a carrot or stick of celery instead of brushing
35. The ducts of the _____ glands open into the floor of the mouth.
    A. Sublingual
    B. Submandibular
    C. Parotid
    D. Carotid
36. The volume of saliva secreted per day is about:
    A. One half pint
    B. One pint
    C. One liter
    D. One gallon
37. Mumps are an infection of the:
    A. Parotid gland
    B. Sublingual gland
    C. Submandibular gland
    D. Tonsils
38. Incisors are used during mastication to:
    A. Cut
    B. Piece
    C. Tear
    D. Grind
39. Another name for the third molar is:
    A. Central incisor
    B. Wisdom tooth
    C. Canine
    D. Lateral incisor
40. After food has been chewed, it is formed into a small rounded mass called a:
    A. Moat
    B. Chyme
    C. Bolus
    D. Protease

▶ *If you have had difficulty with this section, review pages 364-368.*

PHARYNX
ESOPHAGUS
STOMACH

Fill in the blanks.

The (41) _____ is a tubelike structure that functions as part of both respiratory and digestive systems. It connects the mouth with the (42) _____. The esophagus serves as a passageway for movement of food from the pharynx to the (43) _____. Food enters the stomach by passing through the muscular (44) _____ _____ at the end of the esophagus. Contraction of the stomach mixes the food thoroughly with the gastric juices and breaks it down into a semisolid mixture called (45) _____.
The three divisions of the stomach are the (46) _____, the
(47) _____, and the (48) _____.
Food is held in the stomach by the (49) _____ _____ muscle long enough for partial digestion to occur. After food has been in the stomach for approximately 3 hours, the chyme will enter the (50) _____ _____.

Match the term with the correct definition.

A. Esophagus
B. Chyme
C. Peristalsis
D. Rugae
E. Triple therapy

F. Greater curvature
G. Hiatal hernia
H. Tagamet
I. Acid indigestion
J. Lesser curvature

_____ 51. Stomach folds
_____ 52. Upper right border of stomach
_____ 53. Condition that may result in backward movement or reflux of stomach contents into the lower portion of the esophagus
_____ 54. 10-inch passageway
_____ 55. Drug used to treat GERD
_____ 56. Semisolid mixture of stomach contents
_____ 57. Muscle contractions of the digestive system
_____ 58. Used to heal ulcers and prevent recurrences
_____ 59. Heartburn
_____ 60. Lower left border of stomach

▷ *If you have had difficulty with this section, review pages 368-373.*

SMALL INTESTINE
LIVER AND GALLBLADDER
PANCREAS

Circle the best answer.

61. Which one is *not* part of the small intestine?
    A. Jejunum
    B. Ileum
    C. Cecum
    D. Duodenum

62. Which one of the following structures does *not* increase the surface area of the intestine for absorption?
    A. Plicae
    B. Rugae
    C. Villi
    D. Brush border

63. The union of the cystic duct and hepatic duct form the:
    A. Common bile duct
    B. Major duodenal papilla
    C. Minor duodenal papilla
    D. Pancreatic duct

64. Obstruction of the _____ will lead to jaundice.
    A. Hepatic duct
    B. Pancreatic duct
    C. Cystic duct
    D. None of the above

65. Each villus in the intestine contains a lymphatic vessel or _____ that serves to absorb lipid or fat materials from the chyme.
    A. Plica
    B. Lacteal
    C. Villa
    D. Microvilli

66. The middle third of the duodenum contains the:
    A. Islets
    B. Fundus
    C. Body
    D. Rugae
    E. Major duodenal papilla

67. Most gastric and duodenal ulcers result from infection with the bacterium:
    A. Biaxin
    B. Metronidazole
    C. Prilosec
    D. Helicobacter pylori

68. The liver is an:
    A. Enzyme
    B. Endocrine organ
    C. Endocrine gland
    D. Exocrine gland
69. Fats in chyme stimulate the secretion of the hormone:
    A. Lipase
    B. Cholecystokinin
    C. Protease
    D. Amylase
70. The largest gland in the body is the:
    A. Pituitary
    B. Thyroid
    C. Liver
    D. Thymus

 If you have had difficulty with this section, review pages 370-374.

LARGE INTESTINE
APPENDIX
PERITONEUM

If the statement is true, write "T" in the answer blank. If the statement is false, correct the statement by circling the incorrect term and writing the correct term in the answer blank.

_____ 71. Bacteria in the large intestine are responsible for the synthesis of vitamin E needed for normal blood clotting.
_____ 72. Villi in the large intestine absorb salts and water.
_____ 73. If waste products pass rapidly through the large intestine, constipation results.
_____ 74. The ileocecal valve opens into the sigmoid colon.
_____ 75. The splenic flexure is the bend between the ascending colon and the transverse colon.
_____ 76. The splenic colon is the **S**-shaped segment that terminates in the rectum.
_____ 77. The appendix serves no important digestive function in humans.
_____ 78. For patients with suspected appendicitis, a physician will often evaluate the appendix by a digital rectal examination.
_____ 79. The visceral layer of the peritoneum lines the abdominal cavity.
_____ 80. The greater omentum is shaped like a fan and serves to anchor the small intestine to the posterior abdominal wall.

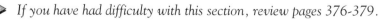 *If you have had difficulty with this section, review pages 376-379.*

DIGESTION
ABSORPTION
METABOLISM

Circle the best answer.

81. Which one of the following substances does *not* contain any enzymes?
    A. Saliva
    B. Bile
    C. Gastric juice
    D. Pancreatic juice
    E. Intestinal juice

82. Which one of the following is a simple sugar?
    A. Maltose
    B. Sucrose
    C. Lactose
    D. Glucose
    E. Starch

83. Cane sugar is the same as:
    A. Maltose
    B. Lactose
    C. Sucrose
    D. Glucose
    E. None of the above

84. Most of the digestion of carbohydrates takes place in the:
    A. Mouth
    B. Stomach
    C. Small intestine
    D. Large intestine

85. Fats are broken down into:
    A. Amino acids
    B. Simple sugars
    C. Fatty acids
    D. Disaccharides

 If you have had difficulty with this section, review page 380.

CHEMICAL DIGESTION

86. Fill in the blank areas on the chart below.

Digestive Juices and Enzymes	Substance Digested (or Hydrolyzed)	Resulting Product
SALIVA		
1. Amylase	1. _____	1. Maltose
GASTRIC JUICE		
2. Protease (pepsin) plus hydrochloric acid	2. Proteins	2. _____
PANCREATIC JUICE		
3. Protease (trypsin)	3. Proteins (intact or partially digested)	3. _____
4. Lipase	4. _____	4. Fatty acids, monoglycerides, and glycerol
5. Amylase	5. _____	5. Maltose
INTESTINAL JUICE		
6. Peptidases	6. _____	6. Amino acids
7. _____	7. Sucrose	7. Glucose and fructose
8. Lactase	8. _____	8. Glucose and galactose (simple sugars)
9. Maltase	9. Maltose	9. _____

If you have had difficulty with this section, review page 381.

UNSCRAMBLE THE WORDS

87. S L B O U

88. E Y C H M

89. L L A A P P I

90. P M E R T E U I O N

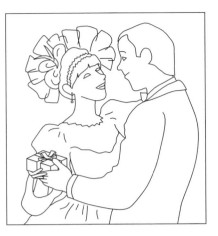

Take the circled letters, unscramble them, and fill in the statement.

What the groom gave his bride after the wedding.

91.

APPLYING WHAT YOU KNOW

92. Mr. Amato was a successful businessman, but he worked too hard and was always under great stress. His doctor cautioned him that if he did not alter his style of living he would be subject to hyperacidity. What could be the resulting condition of hyperacidity?

   _____

93. Baby Shearer has been regurgitating his bottle feeding at every meal. The milk is curdled, but it does not appear to be digested. He has become dehydrated, and so his mother is taking him to the pediatrician. What is a possible diagnosis from your textbook reading?

   _____

94. Mr. Attanas has gained a great deal of weight suddenly. He also has been noticing that he is sluggish and always tired. What test might his physician order for him and for what reason?

   _____

   _____

95. WORD FIND

Can you find 22 terms from the chapter? Words may be spelled top to bottom, bottom to top, right to left, left to right, or diagonally.

```
X  M  E  T  A  B  O  L  I  S  M  X  X  W
R  S  D  P  E  R  I  S  T  A  L  S  I  S
E  V  A  M  N  O  I  T  S  E  G  I  D  R
E  D  E  E  U  O  Q  T  W  Q  O  H  N  Q
Q  Z  H  S  R  N  I  N  T  F  E  C  E  S
D  H  R  E  C  C  I  T  K  C  J  A  P  E
Q  W  R  N  A  T  N  V  P  Y  R  M  P  C
O  C  A  T  N  R  B  A  P  R  H  O  A  I
U  Y  I  E  O  W  T  A  P  A  O  T  W  D
B  O  D  R  L  N  P  B  F  Q  J  S  V  N
N  T  S  Y  F  I  S  L  U  M  E  E  B  U
W  G  J  A  L  U  V  U  N  R  N  W  O  A
Q  S  N  L  X  D  U  O  D  E  N  U  M  J
H  C  A  V  I  T  Y  M  U  C  O  S  A  D
Y  E  A  A  P  H  V  W  S  V  C  Q  J  C
```

Absorption   Emulsify   Mucosa
Appendix   Feces   Pancreas
Cavity   Fundus   Papillae
Crown   Heartburn   Peristalsis
Dentin   Jaundice   Stomach
Diarrhea   Mastication   Uvula
Digestion   Mesentery
Duodenum   Metabolism

DID YOU KNOW?

The liver performs over 500 functions and produces over 1000 enzymes to handle the chemical conversions necessary for survival.

DIGESTIVE SYSTEM

Fill in the crossword puzzle.

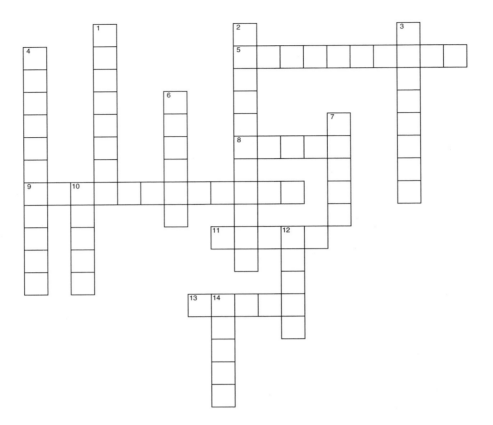

Across

5. Movement of digested food from intestine to blood
8. Semisolid mixture
9. Inflammation of the appendix
11. Rounded mass of food
13. Stomach folds

Down

1. Yellowish skin discoloration
2. Process of chewing
3. Fluid stools
4. Movement of food through the digestive tract
6. Vomitus
7. Waste product of digestion
10. Intestinal folds
12. Open wound in digestive area acted on by acid juices
14. Prevents food from entering nasal cavities

CHECK YOUR KNOWLEDGE

Multiple Choice

Circle the correct answer.

1. During the process of digestion, *stored* bile is poured into the duodenum by which of the following?
   A. Gallbladder
   B. Liver
   C. Pancreas
   D. Spleen

2. The _____ is the portion of the alimentary canal that mixes food with gastric juice and breaks it down into a mixture called chyme.
   A. Gallbladder
   B. Small intestine
   C. Stomach
   D. Large intestine

3. What is the middle portion of the small intestine called?
   A. Jejunum
   B. Ileum
   C. Duodenum
   D. Cecum

4. The crown of the tooth is covered externally with which of the following?
   A. Cementum
   B. Enamel
   C. Dentin
   D. Pulp

5. What is the layer of tissue that forms the outermost covering of organs found in the digestive tract called?
   A. Mucosa
   B. Serosa
   C. Submucosa
   D. Muscularis

6. Duodenal ulcers appear in which of the following?
   A. Stomach
   B. Small intestine
   C. Large intestine
   D. Esophagus

7. What is an extension of the peritoneum that is shaped like a giant, pleated fan?
   A. Omentum
   B. Mesentery
   C. Peritoneal cavity
   D. Ligament

8. Protein digestion begins in the:
   A. Esophagus
   B. Small intestine
   C. Stomach
   D. Large Intestine

9. The enzyme pepsin is concerned primarily with the digestion of which of the following?
   A. Sugars
   B. Starches
   C. Proteins
   D. Fats
10. The enzyme amylase converts which of the following?
    A. Starches to sugars
    B. Sugars to starches
    C. Proteins to amino acids
    D. Fatty acids and glycerols to fats

Completion

Complete the following statements using the terms listed below:

A. Ileum
B. Amylase
C. Muscularis
D. Metabolism
E. Cholecystokinin
F. Molars
G. Cardiac sphincter
H. Digestion
I. Incisors
J. Greater omentum
K. Absorption
L. Adventitia

M. Pyloric sphincter
N. Sigmoid colon
O. Canines
P. Amino acids
Q. Duodenum
R. Jejunum
S. Premolars
T. Mucosa
U. Submucosa
V. Cecum
W. Bile
X. Serosa

11. The **S**-shaped portion of the colon is called the _____.
12. The portion of the peritoneum that descends from the stomach and the transverse colon to form a lacy apron of fat over the intestines is called the _____ _____.
13. The "building blocks" of protein molecules are _____ _____.
14. The small intestine is made up of three sections called the _____, _____, and the _____.
15. Fats that enter into the digestive tract are emulsified when they are acted upon by a substance called _____.
16. Foods undergo three kinds of processing in the body: _____, _____, and _____.
17. Fats in the chyme stimulate the secretion of _____, which stimulates contraction of the gallbladder to release bile.
18. The four tissue layers that make up the wall of the digestive tract are _____, _____, _____, and _____.
19. Food enters the stomach by passing through a muscular structure at the end of the esophagus. This structure is called the _____ _____.
20. The four major types of teeth found in the human mouth are _____, _____, _____, and _____.

Digestive Organs

1. _____

2. _____

3. _____

4. _____

5. _____

6. _____

7. _____

8. _____

9. _____

10. _____

11. _____

12. _____

13. _____

14. _____

15. _____

16. _____

17. _____

18. _____

19. _____

20. _____

21. _____

22. _____

23. _____

24. _____

25. _____

26. _____

27. _____

28. _____

29. _____

30. _____

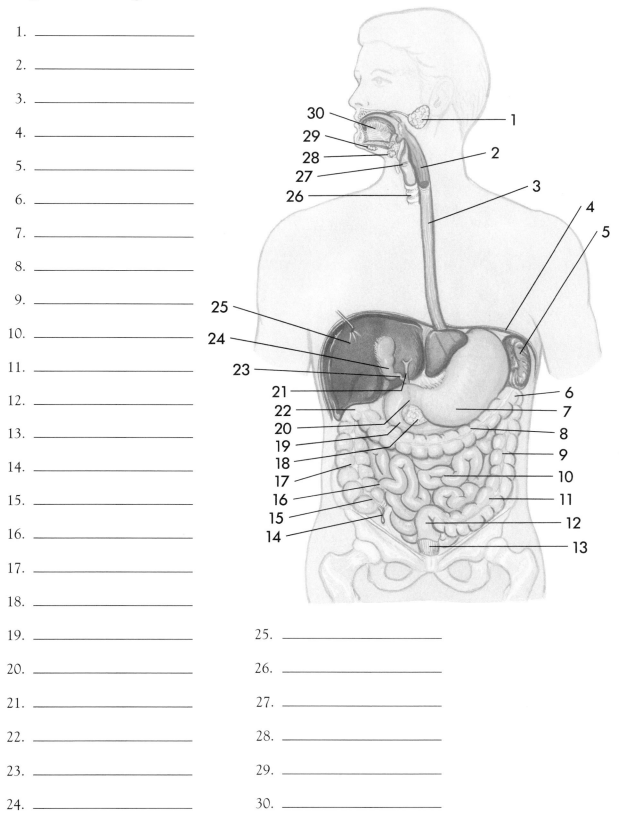

Tooth

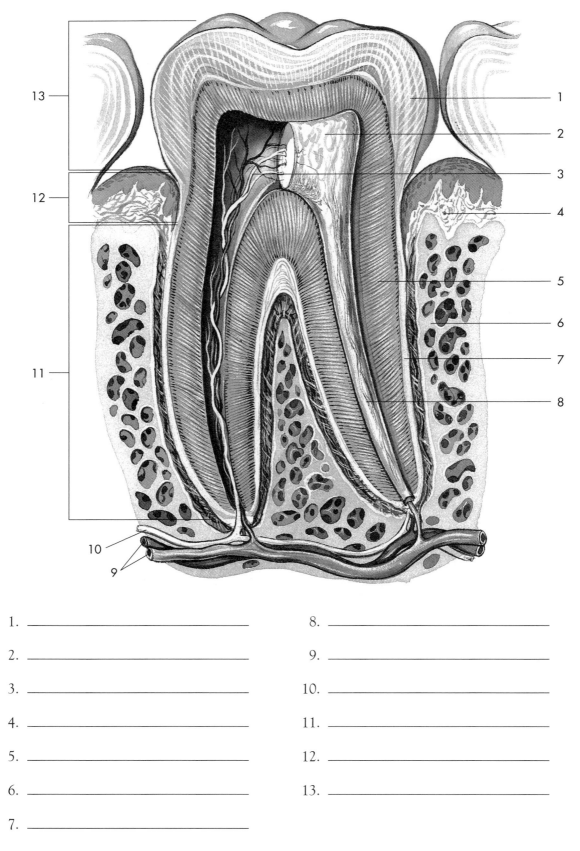

1. _____
2. _____
3. _____
4. _____
5. _____
6. _____
7. _____

8. _____
9. _____
10. _____
11. _____
12. _____
13. _____

The Salivary Glands

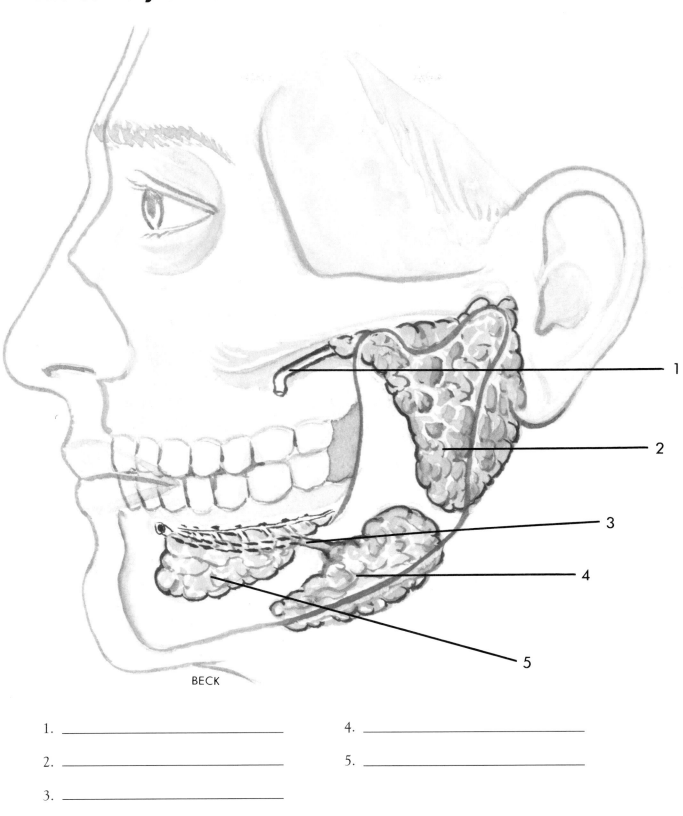

BECK

1. _____   4. _____

2. _____   5. _____

3. _____

Stomach

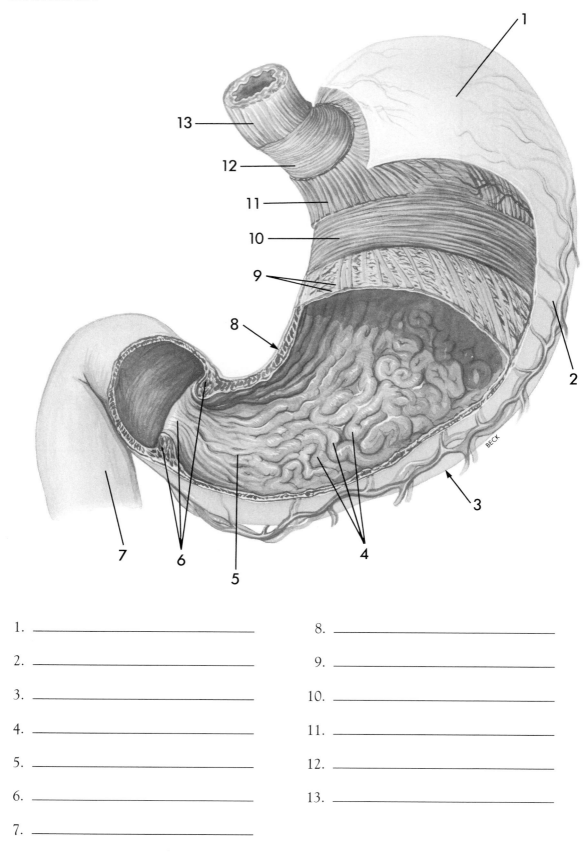

BECK

1. _____

2. _____

3. _____

4. _____

5. _____

6. _____

7. _____

8. _____

9. _____

10. _____

11. _____

12. _____

13. _____

196   Chapter 14: The Digestive System

Gallbladder and Bile Ducts

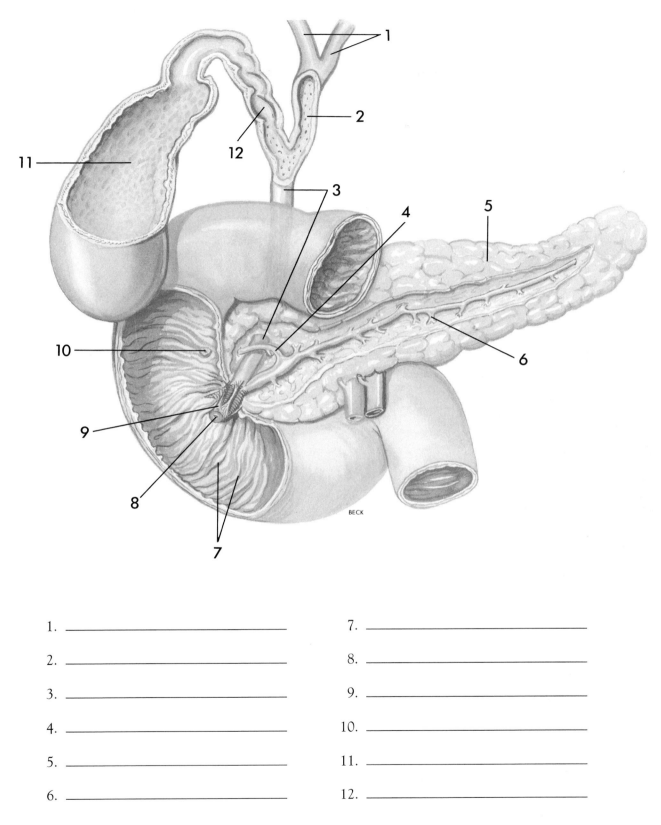

1. _____
2. _____
3. _____
4. _____
5. _____
6. _____

7. _____
8. _____
9. _____
10. _____
11. _____
12. _____

Chapter 14: The Digestive System   197

The Small Intestine

SEGMENT OF JEJUNUM

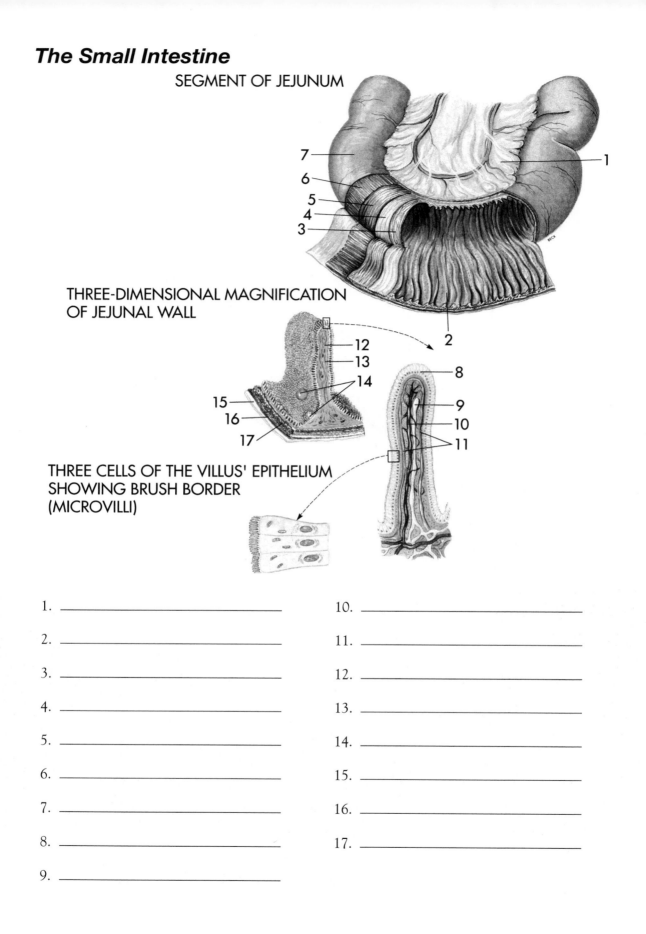

THREE-DIMENSIONAL MAGNIFICATION
OF JEJUNAL WALL

THREE CELLS OF THE VILLUS' EPITHELIUM
SHOWING BRUSH BORDER
(MICROVILLI)

1. _____

2. _____

3. _____

4. _____

5. _____

6. _____

7. _____

8. _____

9. _____

10. _____

11. _____

12. _____

13. _____

14. _____

15. _____

16. _____

17. _____

The Large Intestine

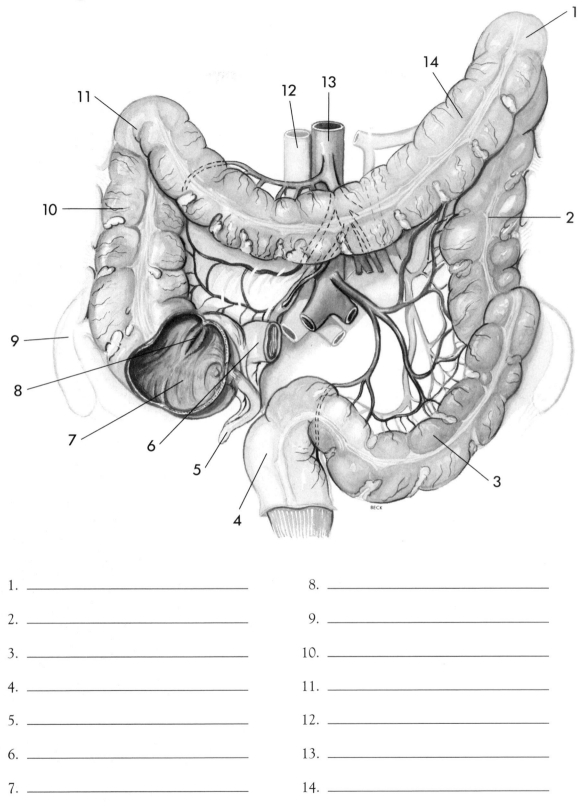

1. _____
2. _____
3. _____
4. _____
5. _____
6. _____
7. _____
8. _____
9. _____
10. _____
11. _____
12. _____
13. _____
14. _____

CHAPTER 15 Nutrition and Metabolism

Most of us love to eat, but do the foods we enjoy provide us with the basic food types necessary for good nutrition? The body, a finely tuned machine, requires a balance of carbohydrates, fats, proteins, vitamins, and minerals to function properly. These nutrients must be digested, absorbed, and circulated to cells constantly to accommodate the numerous activities that occur throughout the body. The use the body makes of foods once these processes are completed is called "metabolism."

The liver plays a major role in the metabolism of food. It helps maintain a normal blood glucose level, removes toxins from the blood, processes blood immediately after it leaves the gastrointestinal tract, and initiates the first steps of protein and fat metabolism.

This chapter also discusses basal metabolic rate (BMR). The BMR is the rate at which food is catabolized under basal conditions. This test and the measurement of the amount of protein-bound iodine (PBI) are indirect measures of thyroid gland functioning. The total metabolic rate (TMR) is the amount of energy, expressed in calories, used by the body each day.

Finally, maintaining a constant body temperature is a function of the hypothalamus and a challenge for the metabolic factors of the body. Review of this chapter is necessary to provide you with an understanding of the "fuel" or nutrition necessary to maintain your complex homeostatic machine—the body.

TOPICS FOR REVIEW

Before progressing to Chapter 16, you should be able to define and contrast catabolism and anabolism. Your review should include the metabolic roles of carbohydrates, fats, proteins, vitamins, and minerals. Your study should conclude with an understanding of the basal metabolic rate and the physiological mechanisms that regulate body temperature.

THE ROLE OF THE LIVER

Fill in the blanks.

The liver plays an important role in the mechanical digestion of lipids because it secretes
(1) _____. It also produces two of the plasma proteins that play an essential role in
blood clotting: (2) _____ and (3) _____. Additionally, liver cells
store several substances, notably vitamins A and D and (4) _____. Finally, the liver
is assisted by a unique structural feature of the blood vessels that supply it. This arrangement, known
as the (5) _____ _____ _____, allows toxins to
be removed from the bloodstream before nutrients are distributed throughout the body.

NUTRIENT METABOLISM

Match the term on the left with the proper selection on the right.

_____	6. Used if cells have inadequate amounts of glucose to catabolize	A. Carbohydrates
_____	7. Preferred energy food	B. Fats
_____	8. Amino acids	C. Proteins
_____	9. Fat soluble	D. Vitamins
_____	10. Required for nerve conduction	E. Minerals
_____	11. Glycolysis	
_____	12. Inorganic elements found naturally in the earth	
_____	13. Pyruvic acid	

Circle the one that does not belong.

14. Glycolysis	Citric acid cycle	ATP	Bile
15. Adipose	Amino acids	Triglycerides	Glycerol
16. A	D	M	K
17. Iron	Proteins	Amino acids	Essential
18. Hydrocortisone	Insulin	Growth hormone	Epinephrine
19. Sodium	Calcium	Zinc	Folic acid
20. Thiamine	Niacin	Ascorbic acid	Riboflavin

 If you have had difficulty with this section, review pages 390-394.

METABOLIC RATES
BODY TEMPERATURE

Circle the correct answer.

21. The rate at which food is catabolized under basal conditions is the:
    A. TMR
    B. PBI
    C. BMR
    D. ATP

22. The total amount of energy used by the body per day is the:
    A. TMR
    B. PBI
    C. BMR
    D. ATP
23. Over _____ of the energy released from food molecules during catabolism is converted to heat rather than transferred to ATP.
    A. 20%
    B. 40%
    C. 60%
    D. 80%
24. Maintaining thermoregulation is a function of the:
    A. Thalamus
    B. Hypothalamus
    C. Thyroid
    D. Parathyroids
25. Transfer of heat energy to the skin and then to the external environment is known as:
    A. Radiation
    B. Conduction
    C. Convection
    D. Evaporation
26. A flow of heat waves away from the blood is known as:
    A. Radiation
    B. Conduction
    C. Convection
    D. Evaporation
27. A transfer of heat energy to air that is continually flowing away from the skin is known as:
    A. Radiation
    B. Conduction
    C. Convection
    D. Evaporation
28. Heat that is absorbed by the process of water vaporization is called:
    A. Radiation
    B. Conduction
    C. Convection
    D. Evaporation
29. A/an _____ is the amount of energy needed to raise the temperature of 1 gram of water 1° centigrade.
    A. Calorie
    B. Kilocalorie
    C. ATP
    D. BMR

 If you have had difficulty with this section, review pages 394-398.

UNSCRAMBLE THE WORDS

30. LRIEV

31. TAOBALICMS

32. OMNIA

33. YPURCVI

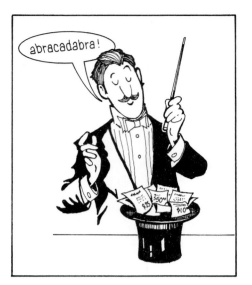

abracadabra!

Take the circled letters, unscramble them, and fill in the statement.

How the magician paid his bills.

34.

APPLYING WHAT YOU KNOW

35. Dr. LaGasse was concerned about Deborrah. Her daily food intake provided fewer calories than her TMR. If this trend continues, what will be the result? If it continues over a long period of time, what eating disorder might Deborrah develop?

_____

_____

36. Mrs. Bishop was experiencing fatigue and a blood test revealed that she was slightly anemic. What mineral will her doctor most likely prescribe? What dietary sources might you suggest that she emphasize in her daily intake?

_____

_____

37. Mr. Thivierge was training daily for an upcoming marathon. Three days before the 25 mile event, he suddenly quit his daily routine of jogging and switched to a diet high in carbohydrates. Why did Mr. Thivierge suddenly switch his routine of training?

_____

_____

204   Chapter 15: Nutrition and Metabolism

38. WORD FIND

Can you find 18 terms from this chapter? Words may be spelled top to bottom, bottom to top, right to left, left to right, or diagonally.

```
C C C B W E F F L J V G G S
A T N L W E U O Z I E L I B
R K K P Z F R I T P O Y K L
B Q M I N E R A L S J C C P
O S S N C X M I D B D O W P
H S I Y O I T X H I N L S N
Y E L N N I K W W D S Y N S
D G O S O W T I U E H S C N
R M B Y T I W C Z N N I A A
A R A Q W A T B E I G S J M
T E T F N I F A E V E W T Y
E V A P O R A T I O N D T E
S I C N E S O P I D A O F E
H L Y K I R E B V P A H C J
I W E E P A D F T E A R G G
```

ATP	Conduction	Liver
Adipose	Convection	Minerals
BMR	Evaporation	Proteins
Bile	Fats	Radiation
Carbohydrates	Glycerol	TMR
Catabolism	Glycolysis	Vitamins

DID YOU KNOW?

The amount of energy required to raise a 200-pound man 15 feet is about the amount of energy in one large calorie.

NUTRITION/METABOLISM

Fill in the crossword puzzle.

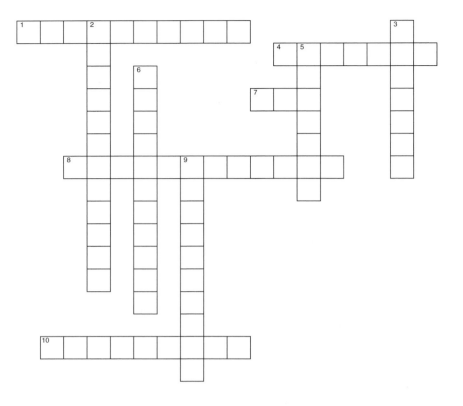

Across

1. Breaks food molecules down releasing stored energy
4. Amount of energy needed to raise the temperature of 1 gram of water 1° centigrade
7. Rate of metabolism when a person is lying down but awake (abbreviation)
8. A series of reactions that join glucose molecules together to form glycogen
10. Builds food molecules into complex substances

Down

2. Occurs when food molecules enter cells and undergo many chemical changes there
3. Organic molecule needed in small quantities for normal metabolism throughout the body
5. Oxygen-using
6. A unit of measure for heat, also known as a large calorie
9. Takes place in the cytoplasm of a cell and changes glucose to pyruvic acid

CHECK YOUR KNOWLEDGE

Multiple Choice

Circle the correct answer.

1. What is the process by which pyruvic acid is broken down into carbon dioxide called?
   A. Glycogenesis
   B. Citric acid cycle
   C. Glycolysis
   D. Pyruvic acid cycle

2. The anabolism of glucose produces which of the following?
   A. Glycogen
   B. Amino acid
   C. Rennin
   D. Starch

3. Which of the following is a major hormone in the body that aids carbohydrate metabolism?
   A. Oxytocin
   B. Epinephrine
   C. Insulin
   D. Growth hormone

4. The total metabolic rate is which of the following?
   A. The amount of fats we consume in a 24-hour period.
   B. The same as the BMR.
   C. The amount of energy expressed in calories used by the body per day.
   D. Cannot be calculated

5. When your consumption of calories equals your TMR, your weight will do which of the following?
   A. Increase
   B. Remain the same
   C. Fluctuate
   D. Decrease

6. Which of the following is a normal glucose level?
   A. 40 to 80 mg/100 ml blood
   B. 80 to 120 mg/100 ml blood
   C. 100 to 140 mg/100 ml blood
   D. 180 to 220 mg/100 ml blood

7. When glucose is *not* available, the body will next catabolize which of the following energy sources?
   A. Fats
   B. Proteins
   C. Minerals
   D. Vitamins

8. Maintaining the homeostasis of the body temperature is the responsibility of which of the following?
   A. Hypothalamus
   B. Environmental condition in which we live
   C. Circulatory system
   D. None of the above

9. The liver plays an important role in the mechanical digestion of lipids because it secretes:
   A. Glucose molecules
   B. Bile
   C. Glycogen
   D. Citric acid
10. What is the primary molecule the body usually breaks down as an energy source?
   A. Amino acid
   B. Pepsin
   C. Maltose
   D. Glucose

Completion

Complete the following statements using the terms listed below. Some words may be used more than once.

A. Vitamins	G. ATP
B. Insulin	H. Sodium
C. Carbohydrates	I. Proteins
D. Fats	J. Citric acid cycle
E. Glycolysis	K. Calcium
F. Heat	L. Glycogen loading

11. Proper nutrition requires the balance of the three basic food types: _____, _____, and _____.
12. The process that changes glucose to pyruvic acid is called _____.
13. Once glucose has been changed to pyruvic acid, another process in which pyruvic acid is changed to carbon dioxide takes place. This reaction is known as the _____ _____ _____.
14. A direct source of energy for doing cellular work is _____.
15. The only hormone that lowers blood glucose level is _____.
16. When cells have an inadequate amount of glucose to catabolize, they will catabolize _____.
17. Some athletes consume large amounts of carbohydrates 2 to 3 days before an athletic event to store glycogen in skeletal muscles. This practice is called _____ _____.
18. Organic molecules needed in small amounts for normal metabolism are _____.
19. Two minerals necessary for nerve conduction and contraction of muscle fibers are _____ and _____.
20. During catabolism, food molecules are converted to _____ rather than being transported to ATP.

CHAPTER **16**   # The Urinary System

Living produces wastes. Wherever people live or work or play, wastes accumulate. To keep these areas healthy, there must be a method of disposing of these wastes such as a sanitation department.

Wastes accumulate in your body also. The conversion of food and gases into substances and energy necessary for survival results in waste products. A large percentage of these wastes is removed by the urinary system.

Two vital organs, the kidneys, cleanse the blood of the many waste products that are continually produced as a result of the metabolism of food in the body cells. They eliminate these wastes in the form of urine.

Urine formation is the result of three processes: filtration, reabsorption, and secretion. These processes occur in successive portions of the microscopic units of the kidneys known as nephrons. The amount of urine produced by the nephrons is controlled primarily by the hormones ADH and aldosterone.

After urine is produced it is drained from the renal pelvis by the ureters to flow into the bladder. The bladder then stores the urine until it is voided through the urethra.

If waste products are allowed to accumulate in the body they soon become poisonous, a condition called uremia. A knowledge of the urinary system is necessary to understand how the body rids itself of waste and avoids toxicity.

TOPICS FOR REVIEW

Before progressing to Chapter 17, you should have an understanding of the structure and function of the organs of the urinary system. Your review should include knowledge of the nephron and its role in urine production. Your study should conclude with a review of the three main processes involved in urine production and the mechanisms that control urine volume.

KIDNEYS

Circle the correct answer.

1. The outermost portion of the kidney is known as the:
   A. Medulla
   B. Papilla
   C. Pelvis
   D. Pyramid
   E. Cortex

2. The sac-like structure that surrounds the glomerulus is the:
   A. Renal pelvis
   B. Calyx
   C. Bowman's capsule
   D. Cortex
   E. None of the above

3. The renal corpuscle is made up of the:
   A. Bowman's capsule and proximal convoluted tubule
   B. Glomerulus and proximal convoluted tubule
   C. Bowman's capsule and the distal convoluted tubule
   D. Glomerulus and the distal convoluted tubule
   E. Bowman's capsule and the glomerulus

4. Which of the following functions is *not* performed by the kidneys?
   A. Maintenance of homeostasis
   B. Removal of wastes from the blood
   C. Production of ADH
   D. Removal of electrolytes from the blood

5. _____ percent of the glomerular filtrate is reabsorbed.
   A. Twenty
   B. Forty
   C. Seventy-five
   D. Eighty-five
   E. Ninety-nine

6. The glomerular filtration rate is _____ ml per minute.
   A. 1.25
   B. 12.5
   C. 125.0
   D. 1250.0
   E. None of the above

7. Glucose is reabsorbed in the:
   A. Loop of Henle
   B. Proximal convoluted tubule
   C. Distal convoluted tubule
   D. Glomerulus
   E. None of the above

8. Reabsorption does *not* occur in the:
   A. Loop of Henle
   B. Proximal convoluted tubule
   C. Distal convoluted tubule
   D. Collecting tubules
   E. Calyx

9. The greater the amount of salt intake, the:
   A. Less salt excreted in the urine
   B. More salt is reabsorbed
   C. More salt excreted in the urine
   D. None of the above

10. Which one of the following substances is secreted by diffusion?
    A. Sodium ions
    B. Certain drugs
    C. Ammonia
    D. Hydrogen ions
    E. Potassium ions

11. Which of the following statements about ADH is *not* true?
    A. It is stored by the pituitary gland.
    B. It makes the collecting tubules less permeable to water.
    C. It makes the distal convoluted tubules more permeable.
    D. It is produced by the hypothalamus.

12. Which of the following statements about aldosterone is *not* true?
    A. It is secreted by the adrenal cortex.
    B. It is a water-retaining hormone.
    C. It is a salt-retaining hormone.
    D. All of the above are correct

Choose the correct term and write the letter in the space next to the appropriate definition below.

A. Medulla
B. Cortex
C. Pyramids
D. Papilla
E. Pelvis
F. Calyx
G. Nephrons

H. Uremia
I. Proteinuria
J. Bowman's capsule
K. Glomerulus
L. Loop of Henle
M. CAPD
N. Glycosuria

_____ 13. Functioning unit of the urinary system
_____ 14. Abnormally large amounts of plasma proteins in the urine
_____ 15. Uremic poisoning
_____ 16. Outer part of kidney
_____ 17. Together with Bowman's capsule forms renal corpuscle
_____ 18. Division of the renal pelvis
_____ 19. Cup-shaped top of a nephron
_____ 20. Innermost end of a pyramid
_____ 21. Extension of proximal tubule
_____ 22. Triangular-shaped divisions of the medulla of the kidney
_____ 23. Used in the treatment of renal failure
_____ 24. Inner portion of kidney

If you have had difficulty with this section, review pages 403-413.

URETERS
URINARY BLADDER
URETHRA

Indicate which organ is identified by the following descriptions by writing the appropriate letter in the answer blank.

      A. Ureters   B. Bladder   C. Urethra

_____ 25. Rugae
_____ 26. Lower-most part of urinary tract
_____ 27. Lining membrane richly supplied with sensory nerve endings
_____ 28. Lies behind pubic symphysis
_____ 29. Dual function in male
_____ 30. 11/2 inches long in female
_____ 31. Drains renal pelvis
_____ 32. Surrounded by prostate in male
_____ 33. Elastic fibers and involuntary muscle fibers
_____ 34. 10 to 12 inches long
_____ 35. Trigone

Fill in the blanks.

36. _____ _____ is the description of the pain caused by the passage of a kidney stone.
37. The urinary tract is lined with _____ _____.
38. Another name for kidney stones is _____ _____.
39. A technique that uses _____ to pulverize stones, thus avoiding surgery, is being used to treat kidney stones.
40. The passage of a tube through the urethra into the bladder for the removal of urine is known as _____.
41. The _____ _____ is the basinlike upper end of the ureter located inside the kidney.
42. In the male, the urethra as a passageway for both urine and _____.
43. The external opening of the urethra is the _____ _____.

 If you have had difficulty with this section, review pages 412-416.

MICTURITION

Fill in the blanks.

The terms (44) _____, (45) _____, and (46) _____ all refer to the passage of urine from the body or the emptying of the bladder. The sphincters guard the bladder. The (47) _____ _____ sphincter is located at the bladder (48) _____ and is involuntary. The external urethral sphincter circles the (49) _____ and is under (50) _____ control.

As the bladder fills, nervous impulses are transmitted to the spinal cord and an (51) _____ _____ is initiated. Urine then enters the (52) _____ to be eliminated.

Urinary (53) _____ is a condition in which no urine is voided. Urinary (54) _____ is when the kidneys do not produce any urine, but the bladder retains its ability to empty itself. Complete destruction or transection of the sacral cord produces an (55) _____ _____.

 If you have had difficulty with this section, review pages 415-416.

UNSCRAMBLE THE WORDS

56. A Y X L C

[ ][ ][ ](◯)[ ][ ]

57. G V N O I D I

[ ][ ](◯)(◯)[ ][ ][ ]

58. A L P A L I P

[ ][ ](◯)[ ][ ][ ](◯)

59. S G U L L O U M R E

[ ][ ][ ](◯)[ ](◯)[ ][ ](◯)

Take the circled letters, unscramble them, and fill in the statement.

What Betty saw while cruising down the Nile.

60.

[ ][ ][ ][ ][ ][ ][ ][ ]

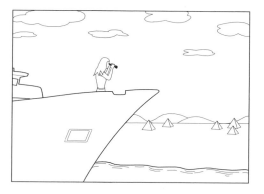

APPLYING WHAT YOU KNOW

61. John suffered from low levels of ADH. What primary urinary symptom would he notice?

_____

62. Bud was in a diving accident and his spinal cord was severed. He was paralyzed from the waist down and as a result was incontinent. His physician was concerned about the continuous residual urine buildup. What was the reason for concern?

_____

63. Mrs. Peace had a prolonged surgical procedure and experienced problems with urinary retention postoperatively. A urinary catheter was inserted into her bladder for the elimination of urine. Several days later, Mrs. Peace developed cystitis. What might be a possible cause?

_____

_____

64. WORD FIND

Can you find 18 terms from this chapter? Words may be spelled top to bottom, bottom to top, right to left, left to right, or diagonally.

```
C  C  C  B  W  E  F  F  L  J  V  G  G  S
A  T  N  L  W  E  U  O  Z  I  E  L  I  B
R  K  K  P  Z  F  R  I  T  P  O  Y  K  L
B  Q  M  I  N  E  R  A  L  S  J  C  C  P
O  S  S  N  C  X  M  I  D  B  D  O  W  P
H  S  I  Y  O  I  T  X  H  I  N  L  S  N
Y  E  L  N  N  I  K  W  W  D  S  Y  N  S
D  G  O  S  O  W  T  I  U  E  H  S  C  N
R  M  B  Y  T  I  W  C  Z  N  N  I  A  A
A  R  A  Q  W  A  T  B  E  I  G  S  J  M
T  E  T  F  N  I  F  A  E  V  E  W  T  Y
E  V  A  P  O  R  A  T  I  O  N  D  T  E
S  I  C  N  E  S  O  P  I  D  A  O  F  E
H  L  Y  K  I  R  E  B  V  P  A  H  C  J
I  W  E  E  P  A  D  F  T  E  A  R  G  G
```

ATP   Conduction   Liver
Adipose   Convection   Minerals
BMR   Evaporation   Proteins
Bile   Fats   Radiation
Carbohydrates   Glycerol   TMR
Catabolism   Glycolysis   Vitamins

DID YOU KNOW?

If the tubules in a kidney were stretched out and untangled, there would be 70 miles of them.

URINARY SYSTEM

Fill in the crossword puzzle.

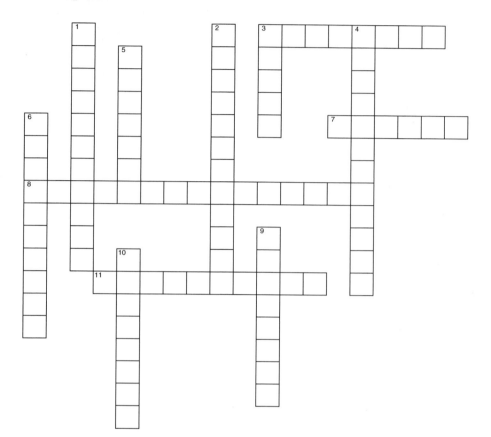

Across

3. Bladder infection
7. Absence of urine
8. Passage of a tube into the bladder to withdraw urine
11. Network of blood capillaries tucked into Bowman's capsule

Down

1. Urination
2. Ultrasound generator used to break up kidney stones
3. Division of the renal pelvis
4. Voiding involuntarily
5. Area on posterior bladder wall free of rugae
6. Glucose in the urine
9. Large amount of urine
10. Scanty urine

CHECK YOUR KNOWLEDGE

Multiple Choice

Circle the correct answer.

1. Which of the following is *true* of urinary catheterization?
   A. It can be used to treat retention.
   B. It requires aseptic technique.
   C. It can lead to cystitis.
   D. All of the above

2. Which of the following processes are used by the artificial kidney to remove waste materials from blood?
   A. Pinocytosis
   B. Dialysis
   C. Catheterization
   D. Active transport

3. Failure of the kidneys to remove wastes from the blood will result in which of the following?
   A. Retention
   B. Anuria
   C. Incontinence
   D. Uremia

4. Hydrogen ions are transferred from blood back into the nephron during which of the following processes?
   A. Secretion
   B. Filtration
   C. Reabsorption
   D. All of the above

5. Which of the following conditions would be considered normal in an infant under 2 years of age?
   A. Retention
   B. Cystitis
   C. Incontinence
   D. Anuria

6. Which of the following steps involved in urine formation allows the blood to retain most body nutrients?
   A. Secretion
   B. Filtration
   C. Reabsorption
   D. All of the above

7. Voluntary control of micturition is achieved by the action of which of the following?
   A. Internal urethral sphincter
   B. External urethral sphincter
   C. Trigone
   D. Bladder muscles
8. What is the structure that carries urine from the kidney to the bladder called?
   A. Urethra
   B. Bowman's capsule
   C. Ureter
   D. Renal pelvis
9. What are the capillary loops contained within Bowman's capsule called?
   A. Convoluted tubules
   B. Glomeruli
   C. Limbs of Henle
   D. Collecting ducts
10. The triangular divisions of the medulla of the kidney are known as:
    A. Pyramids
    B. Papillae
    C. Calyces
    D. Nephrons

Matching

Match the term on the left with the proper selection on the right.

_____ 11. Retention		A. Involuntary voiding
_____ 12. Anuria		B. Movement of substance out of the renal tubules and into the blood
_____ 13. Cystitis		C. Absence of urine
_____ 14. Micturition		D. Urination
_____ 15. Oliguria		E. Bladder does not empty
_____ 16. Polyuria		F. Inflammation of the urinary bladder
_____ 17. Incontinence		G. Large amount of protein in urine
_____ 18. Proteinuria		H. Large amount of urine
_____ 19. Suppression		I. Kidneys not producing urine
_____ 20. Reabsorption		J. Scanty amount of urine

Urinary System

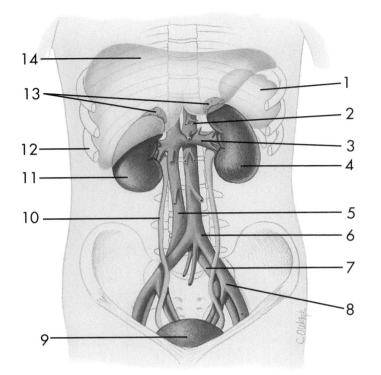

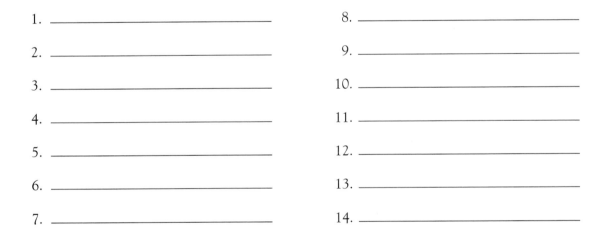

1. _____

2. _____

3. _____

4. _____

5. _____

6. _____

7. _____

8. _____

9. _____

10. _____

11. _____

12. _____

13. _____

14. _____

Kidney

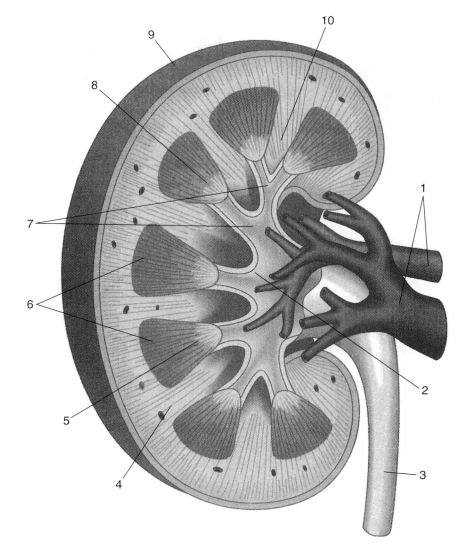

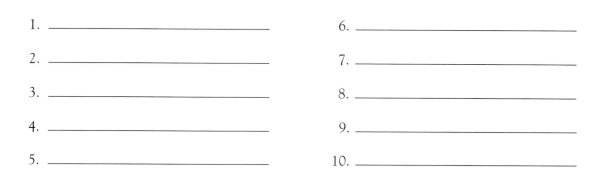

1. _____

2. _____

3. _____

4. _____

5. _____

6. _____

7. _____

8. _____

9. _____

10. _____

Nephron

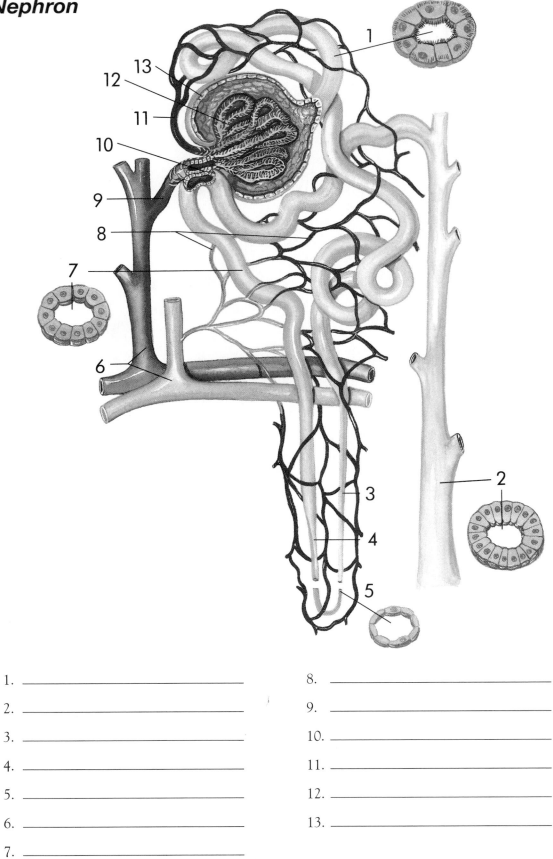

1. _____

2. _____

3. _____

4. _____

5. _____

6. _____

7. _____

8. _____

9. _____

10. _____

11. _____

12. _____

13. _____

CHAPTER **17** # Fluid and Electrolyte Balance

In the very first chapter of the text you learned that survival depends on the body's ability to maintain or restore homeostasis. Specifically, homeostasis means that the body fluids remain constant within very narrow limits. These fluids are classified as either intracellular fluid (ICF) or extracellular fluid (ECF). As the names imply, intracellular fluid lies within the cells and extracellular fluid is located outside the cells. A balance between these two fluids is maintained by certain body mechanisms: (a) the adjustment of fluid output to fluid intake under normal circumstances; (b) the concentration of electrolytes in the extracellular fluid; (c) the capillary blood pressure; and (d) the concentration of proteins in the blood.

Comprehension of how these mechanisms maintain and restore fluid balance is necessary for an understanding of the complexities of homeostasis and its relationship to the survival of the individual.

TOPICS FOR REVIEW

Before progressing to Chapter 18, you should review the types of body fluids and their subdivisions. Your study should include the mechanisms that maintain fluid balance and the nature and importance of electrolytes in body fluids. You should be able to give examples of common fluid imbalances and have an understanding of the role of fluid and electrolyte balance in the maintenance of homeostasis.

BODY FLUIDS

Circle the correct answer.
1. The largest volume of water by far lies (inside or outside) cells.
2. Interstitial fluid is (intracellular or extracellular).
3. Plasma is (intracellular or extracellular).
4. Obese people have a (lower or higher) water content per pound of body weight than thin people.
5. Infants have (more or less) water in comparison to body weight than adults of either sex.
6. There is a rapid (increase or decline) in the proportion of body water to body weight during the first year of life.
7. The female body contains slightly (more or less) water per pound of weight.
8. In general, as age increases, the amount of water per pound of body weight (increases or decreases).
9. Excluding adipose tissue, approximately (55% or 85%) of body weight is water.
10. The term (*"fluid balance"* or *"fluid compartments"*) means that the volumes of ICF, IF, plasma, and the total volume of water in the body all remain relatively constant.

▶ *If you have had difficulty with this section, review pages 424-425.*

MECHANISMS THAT MAINTAIN FLUID BALANCE

Circle the correct answer.
11. Which one of the following is a positively charged ion?
    A. Sodium
    B. Chloride
    C. Phosphate
    D. Bicarbonate
12. Which one of the following is a negatively charged ion?
    A. Sodium
    B. Potassium
    C. Calcium
    D. Chloride
13. The most abundant electrolytes in the blood plasma are:
    A. NaCl
    B. KMg
    C. HCO3
    D. HPO4
    E. CaPO4
14. If the blood sodium concentration increases, then blood volume will:
    A. Increase
    B. Decrease
    C. Remain the same
    D. None of the above

15. The smallest amount of water comes from:
    A. Water in foods that are eaten
    B. Ingested liquids
    C. Water formed from catabolism
    D. None of the above
16. The greatest amount of water lost from the body is from the:
    A. Lungs
    B. Skin, by diffusion
    C. Skin, by sweat
    D. Feces
    E. Kidneys
17. Which one of the following is *not* a major factor that influences extracellular and intracellular fluid volumes?
    A. The concentration of electrolytes in the extracellular fluid
    B. The capillary blood pressure
    C. The concentration of proteins in blood
    D. All of the above are major factors
18. The type of fluid output that changes the most is:
    A. Water loss in the feces
    B. Water loss across the skin
    C. Water loss via the lungs
    D. Water loss in the urine
    E. None of the above
19. The chief regulators of sodium within the body is(are) the:
    A. Lungs
    B. Sweat glands
    C. Kidneys
    D. Large intestine
    E. None of the above
20. Which of the following is *not* true?
    A. Fluid output must equal fluid intake.
    B. ADH controls salt reabsorption in the kidney.
    C. Water follows sodium.
    D. Renal tubule regulation of salt and water is the most important factor in determining urine volume.
21. Diuretics work on all but which one of the following?
    A. Proximal tubule
    B. Loop of Henle
    C. Distal tubule
    D. Collecting ducts
    E. Diuretics work on all of the above
22. Of all the sodium-containing secretions, the one with the largest volume is:
    A. Saliva
    B. Gastric secretions
    C. Bile
    D. Pancreatic juice
    E. Intestinal secretions

23. The higher the capillary blood pressure, the _____ the amount of interstitial fluid.
    A. Smaller
    B. Larger
    C. There is no relationship between capillary blood pressure and volume of interstitial fluid
24. An increase in capillary blood pressure will lead to _____ in blood volume.
    A. An increase
    B. A decrease
    C. No change
    D. None of the above
25. Which one of the fluid compartments varies the *most* in volume?
    A. Intracellular
    B. Interstitial
    C. Extracellular
    D. Plasma
26. Which one of the following will *not* cause edema?
    A. Retention of electrolytes in the extracellular fluid
    B. Increase in capillary blood pressure
    C. Burns
    D. Decrease in plasma proteins
    E. All of the above may cause edema

If the statement is true, write "T" in the answer blank. If the statement is false, correct the statement by circling the incorrect term and writing the correct term in the answer blank.

_____ 27. The three sources of fluid intake are the liquids we drink, the foods we eat, and the water formed by the anabolism of foods.
_____ 28. The body maintains fluid balance mainly by changing the volume of urine excreted to match changes in the volume of fluid intake.
_____ 29. Some output of fluid will occur as long as life continues.
_____ 30. Glucose is an example of an electrolyte.
_____ 31. Where sodium goes, water soon follows.
_____ 32. Excess aldosterone leads to hypovolemia.
_____ 33. Diuretics have their effect on glomerular function.
_____ 34. Typical daily intake and output totals should be approximately 1200 ml.
_____ 35. Bile is a sodium-containing internal secretion.
_____ 36. The average daily diet contains about 500 mEq of sodium.

▷ *If you have had difficulty with this section, review pages 425-432.*

FLUID IMBALANCES

Fill in the blanks.

(37) _____ is the fluid imbalance seen most often. In this condition, interstitial fluid volume (38) _____ first, but eventually, if treatment has not been given, intracellular fluid and plasma volumes (39) _____. (40) _____ can also occur, but it is much less common.

Giving (41) _____ _____ too rapidly or in too large amounts can put too heavy a burden on the (42) _____.

 If you have had difficulty with this section, review page 432.

APPLYING WHAT YOU KNOW

43. Mrs. Titus was asked to keep an accurate record of her fluid intake and output. She was concerned because the two did not balance. What is a possible explanation for this?

_____

_____

_____

44. Nurse Briker was caring for a patient who was receiving diuretics. What special nursing implications should be followed for patients on this therapy?

_____

_____

45. WORD FIND

Can you find 12 terms from this chapter? Words may be spelled top to bottom, bottom to top, right to left, left to right, or diagonally.

```
S  T  V  H  O  M  E  O  S  T  A  S  I  S  H
I  E  D  E  M  A  S  Q  A  L  P  U  E  G  L
M  M  L  U  F  L  U  I  D  O  Y  O  I  S  L
W  S  B  E  A  E  C  O  L  D  P  N  I  E  R
L  I  T  A  C  V  S  H  Q  O  C  E  H  B  C
L  L  X  J  L  T  E  A  W  Y  B  V  Q  Q  O
I  O  P  E  A  R  U  C  T  C  A  A  R  I
N  B  H  R  X  S  N  O  I  I  P  R  T  C  N
S  A  O  X  M  G  J  C  L  N  J  T  B  A  H
I  N  X  X  D  V  U  D  E  Y  K  N  Y  O  C
E  A  A  J  Q  D  I  U  R  E  T  I  C  S  X
I  F  C  J  A  M  P  V  E  N  B  E  Y  F  W
V  F  K  T  Q  X  R  M  D  D  S  I  V  O  T
E  T  T  Z  N  T  R  P  X  I  M  L  J  F  I
S  W  Y  A  P  V  Q  N  S  K  T  K  W  B  P
```

Aldosterone	Edema	Imbalance
Anabolism	Electrolyte	Intravenous
Catabolism	Fluid	Ions
Diuretics	Homeostasis	Kidney

DID YOU KNOW?

The best fluid replacement drink is ¼ teaspoon of table salt to 1 quart of water.

FLUID/ELECTROLYTES

Fill in the crossword puzzle.

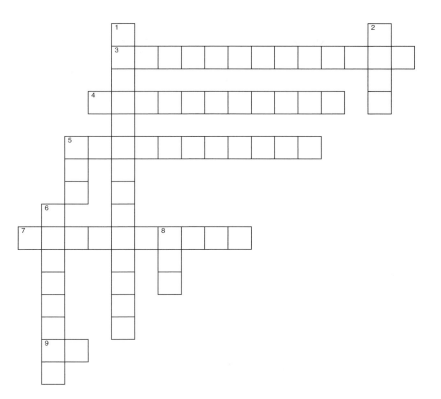

Across

3. Result of rapidly given intravenous fluids
4. Result of large loss of body fluids
5. Compound that dissociates in solution into ions
7. To break up
9. A subdivision of extracellular fluid (abbreviation)

Down

1. Organic substance that does not dissociate in solution
2. Dissociated particles of an electrolyte that carry an electrical charge
5. Fluid outside cells (abbreviation)
6. "Causing urine"
8. Fluid inside cells (abbreviation)

CHECK YOUR KNOWLEDGE

Multiple Choice

Circle the correct answer.

1. Which of the following statements, if any, is *not* true?
   A. The more fat present in the body, the more total water content per unit of weight.
   B. Infants have more water in comparison with body weight than adults.
   C. As age increases, the amount of water per pound of body weight decreases.
   D. All of the above statements are true

2. Avenues of fluid output include which of the following?
   A. Skin
   B. Lungs
   C. Kidneys
   D. All of the above

3. Excessive water loss and fluid imbalance can result from which of the following?
   A. Diarrhea
   B. Vomiting
   C. Severe burns
   D. All of the above

4. What factor is primarily responsible for moving water from interstitial fluid into blood?
   A. Aldosterone secretions
   B. Pressure in blood capillaries
   C. Protein concentration of blood plasma
   D. Antidiuretic hormone secretions

5. What is the chief regulator of sodium levels in body fluids?
   A. Kidney
   B. Intestine
   C. Blood
   D. Lung

6. If blood sodium concentration decreases, what does blood volume do?
   A. Increases
   B. Decreases
   C. Remains the same
   D. None of the above

7. Which of the following is *true* of body water?
   A. It is obtained from the liquids we drink.
   B. It is obtained from the foods we eat.
   C. It is formed by the catabolism of food.
   D. All of the above are true

8. Edema may result from which of the following?
   A. Retention of electrolytes
   B. Decreased blood pressure
   C. Increased concentration of blood plasma proteins
   D. All of the above

9. The most abundant and most important positive plasma ion is which of the following?
   A. Sodium
   B. Chloride
   C. Calcium
   D. Oxygen
10. Which of the following is *true* when extracellular fluid volume decreases?
   A. Aldosterone secretion increases.
   B. Kidney tubule reabsorption of sodium increases.
   C. Urine volume decreases.
   D. All of the above

Completion

Complete the following statements using the terms listed below:

A. Aldosterone	H. Antidiuretic hormone
B. Edema	I. Dehydration
C. Proteins	J. Extracellular fluid
D. Decreases	K. Plasma
E. Diuretic	L. Urine
F. Electrolytes	M. Interstitial fluid
G. Positive	N. Fluid balance

11. Any drug that promotes or stimulates the production of urine is called a _____.
12. The presence of abnormally large amounts of fluid in the intercellular tissue spaces of the body is called _____.
13. Water located outside of cells is called _____ _____. It can be divided into two categories. If it is located in the spaces between the cells, it is called _____ _____. If it is located in the blood vessels, it is called _____.
14. Compounds like sodium chloride that form ions when placed in solution are called _____.
15. When the adrenal cortex increases its secretion of aldosterone, urine volume _____.
16. Most fluids leave the body in the form of _____.
17. When fluid output is greater than fluid intake, _____ occurs.
18. How much water moves into blood from interstitial fluid depends largely on the concentration of _____ present in blood plasma. These substances act as a water-pulling or water-holding force.
19. Urine volume is regulated primarily by a hormone secreted by the posterior lobe of the pituitary gland called _____ _____ and by a hormone secreted by the adrenal gland called _____.
20. Homeostasis of fluids is also known as _____ _____.

CHAPTER **18** Acid-Base Balance

It has been established in previous chapters that an equilibrium between intracellular and extracellular fluid volume must exist for homeostasis to be maintained. Equally important to homeostasis is the chemical acid-base balance of the body fluids. The degree of acidity or alkalinity of a body fluid is expressed in pH value. The neutral point, where a fluid would be neither acid nor alkaline, is pH 7. Increasing acidity is expressed as less than 7, and increasing alkalinity is expressed as greater than 7. Examples of body fluids that are acidic are gastric juice (1.6) and urine (6.0). Blood, on the other hand, is considered alkaline, with a pH of 7.45.

Buffers are substances that prevent a sharp change in the pH of a fluid when an acid or base is added to it. They are one of several mechanisms that are constantly monitoring the pH of fluids in the body. If, for any reason, these mechanisms do not function properly, a pH imbalance occurs. The two kinds of imbalances are known as alkalosis and acidosis.

Maintaining the acid-base balance of body fluids is a matter of vital importance. If this balance varies even slightly, necessary chemical and cellular reactions cannot occur. Your review of this chapter is necessary to understand the delicate fluid balance required for survival.

TOPICS FOR REVIEW

Before progressing to Chapter 19, you should have an understanding of the pH of body fluids and the mechanisms that control the pH of these fluids in the body. Your study should conclude with a review of the metabolic and respiratory types of pH imbalances.

pH OF BODY

Select the correct term from the options given and write the letter in the answer blank.

      A. Acid   B. Base

_____ 1. Lower concentration of hydrogen ions than hydroxide ions

_____ 2. Higher concentration of hydrogen ions than hydroxide ions

_____ 3. Gastric juice

_____ 4. Saliva

_____ 5. Arterial blood

_____ 6. Venous blood

_____ 7. Baking soda

_____ 8. Milk

_____ 9. Ammonia

_____ 10. Egg white

 If you have had difficulty with this section, review page 438.

MECHANISMS THAT CONTROL pH OF BODY FLUIDS
pH IMBALANCES

Circle the correct answer.

11. When carbon dioxide enters the blood, it reacts with the enzyme carbonic anhydrase to form:
    A. Sodium bicarbonate
    B. Water and carbon dioxide
    C. Ammonium chloride
    D. Bicarbonate ion
    E. Carbonic acid

12. The lungs remove _____ liters of carbonic acid each day.
    A. 10.0
    B. 15.0
    C. 20.0
    D. 25.0
    E. 30.0

13. When a buffer reacts with a strong acid, it changes the strong acid to a:
    A. Weak acid
    B. Strong base
    C. Weak base
    D. Water
    E. None of the above

14. Which one of the following is *not* a change in the blood that results from the buffering of fixed acids in tissue capillaries?
    A. The amount of carbonic acid increases slightly.
    B. The amount of bicarbonate in blood decreases.
    C. The hydrogen ion concentration of blood increases slightly.
    D. The blood pH decreases slightly.
    E. All of the above are changes that result from the buffering of fixed acids in tissue capillaries.

15. The most abundant acid in the body:
    A. HCl
    B. Lactic acid
    C. Carbonic acid
    D. Acetic acid
    E. Sulfuric acid
16. The normal ratio of sodium bicarbonate to carbonic acid in arterial blood is:
    A. 5:1
    B. 10:1
    C. 15:1
    D. 20:1
    E. None of the above
17. Which of the following is *not* a consequence of holding your breath?
    A. The amount of carbonic acid in the blood increases.
    B. The blood pH decreases.
    C. The body develops an alkalosis.
    D. No carbon dioxide leaves the body.
18. Which of the following is *not* true of the kidneys?
    A. They can eliminate larger amounts of acid than the lungs.
    B. More bases than acids are usually excreted by the kidneys.
    C. If the kidneys fail, homeostasis of acid-base balance fails.
    D. They are the most effective regulators of blood pH.
19. The pH of the urine may be as low as:
    A. 1.6
    B. 2.5
    C. 3.2
    D. 4.8
    E. 7.4
20. In the distal tubule cells, the product of the reaction aided by carbonic anhydrase is:
    A. Water
    B. Carbon dioxide
    C. Water and carbon dioxide
    D. Hydrogen ions
    E. Carbonic acid
21. In the distal tubule, _____ leaves the tubule cells and enters the blood capillaries.
    A. Carbon dioxide
    B. Water
    C. HCO_3
    D. NaH_2PO_4
    E. $NaHCO_3$

If the statement is true, write "T" in the answer blank. If the statement is false, correct the statement by circling the incorrect term and writing the correct term in the answer blank.

_____ 22. The body has three mechanisms for regulating the pH of its fluids. They are the heart mechanism, the respiratory mechanism, and the urinary mechanism.

_____ 23. Buffers consist of two kinds of substances and are therefore often called duobuffers.

_____ 24. Ordinary baking soda is one of the main buffers of the normally occurring "fixed" acids in the blood.

_____ 25. Some athletes have adopted a technique called bicarbonate loading, whereby they ingest large amounts of sodium bicarbonate ($NaHCO_3$) to counteract the effects of lactic acid buildup.

_____ 26. Anything that causes an excessive increase in respiration will in time produce acidosis.

_____ 27. The lungs are the body's most effective regulator of blood pH.

_____ 28. More acids than bases are usually excreted by the kidneys because more acids than bases usually enter the blood.

_____ 29. Blood levels of sodium bicarbonate can be regulated by the lungs.

_____ 30. Blood levels of carbonic acid can be regulated by the kidneys.

▶ *If you have had difficulty with this section, review pages 439-444.*

pH IMBALANCES
METABOLIC AND RESPIRATORY DISTURBANCES
VOMITING

Write the letter of the correct term on the blank next to the appropriate definition.

A. Metabolic acidosis
B. Metabolic alkalosis
C. Respiratory acidosis
D. Respiratory alkalosis
E. Vomiting

F. Normal saline
G. Uncompensated metabolic acidosis
H. Hyperventilation
I. Hypersalivation
J. Ipecac

_____ 31. Emesis
_____ 32. Result of untreated diabetes
_____ 33. Chloride containing solution
_____ 34. Bicarbonate deficit
_____ 35. Present during emesis
_____ 36. Bicarbonate excess
_____ 37. Rapid breathing
_____ 38. Carbonic acid excess
_____ 39. Carbonic acid deficit
_____ 40. Emetic

▶ *If you have had difficulty with this section, review pages 445-446.*

APPLYING WHAT YOU KNOW

41. Holly is pregnant, and she experienced repeated vomiting episodes for several days. Her doctor became concerned, admitted her to the hospital, and began intravenous administrations of normal saline. How will this help Holly?

_____

_____

_____

42. Cara had a minor bladder infection. She had heard that this is often the result of the urine being less acidic than necessary and that she should drink cranberry juice to correct the acid problem. She had no cranberry juice, so she decided to substitute orange juice. What was wrong with this substitution?

_____

_____

_____

43. Mr. Madden has frequent bouts of hyperacidity of the stomach. Which will assist in neutralizing the acid more promptly, milk or milk of magnesia? Why?

_____

_____

44. WORD FIND

Can you find 18 terms from this chapter? Words may be spelled top to bottom, bottom to top, right to left, left to right, or diagonally.

```
S  I  S  A  T  S  O  E  M  O  H  P  R  G
E  C  N  A  L  A  B  D  I  U  L  F  E  F
T  S  Y  E  N  D  I  K  W  T  I  K  A  J
Y  D  M  N  D  E  J  W  L  P  T  D  J  I
L  D  N  O  L  H  V  W  O  U  H  D  O  I
O  V  E  R  H  Y  D  R  A  T  I  O  N  S
R  E  I  E  E  D  E  M  A  U  R  O  R  Q
T  L  M  T  C  R  U  L  R  F  S  E  O  Y
C  C  U  S  Z  A  W  E  K  A  T  N  I  X
E  O  Z  O  T  T  A  N  A  U  N  M  F
L  F  K  D  P  I  O  I  W  W  Q  L  G  Q
E  N  I  L  C  O  O  H  O  W  S  B  X  S
N  J  X  A  L  N  F  S  U  N  L  J  J  J
O  C  U  V  S  A  L  G  T  I  S  C  Z  X
N  I  Z  L  L  D  Y  X  Q  Q  K  D  C  D
```

ADH	Edema	Nonelectrolytes
Aldosterone	Electrolytes	Output
Anions	Fluid balance	Overhydration
Cations	Homeostasis	Sodium
Dehydration	Intake	Thirst
Diuretic	Kidneys	Water

DID YOU KNOW?

The brain is a greedy 3-lb. organ that demands 17% of all cardiac output and 20% of all available oxygen.

ACID/BASE BALANCE

Fill in the crossword puzzle.

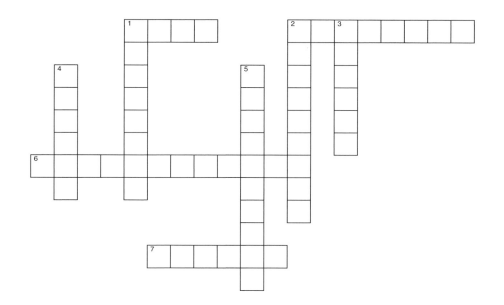

Across

1. Substance with an pH lower than 7.0
2. Acid-base imbalance
6. Result from the excessive metabolism of fats in uncontrolled diabetics (two words)
7. Vomitus

Down

1. Substance with a pH higher than 7.0
2. Serious complication of vomiting
3. Emetic
4. Prevents a sharp change in the pH of fluids
5. Released as a waste product from working muscles (two words)

CHECK YOUR KNOWLEDGE

Multiple Choice

Circle the correct answer.

1. What happens as blood flows through lung capillaries?
   A. Carbonic acid in blood decreases.
   B. Hydrogen ions in blood decrease.
   C. Blood pH increases from venous to arterial blood.
   D. All of the above

2. Which of the following organs is considered to be the *most* effective regulator of blood carbonic acid levels?
   A. Kidneys
   B. Intestines
   C. Lungs
   D. Stomach

3. Which of the following organs is considered to be the *most* effective regulator of blood pH?
   A. Kidneys
   B. Intestines
   C. Lungs
   D. Stomach

4. What is the pH of the blood?
   A. 7.00 to 8.00
   B. 6.25 to 7.45
   C. 7.65 to 7.85
   D. 7.35 to 7.45

5. If the ratio of sodium bicarbonate to carbonate ions is lowered (perhaps 10 to 1) and blood pH is also lowered, what is the condition called?
   A. Uncompensated metabolic acidosis
   B. Uncompensated metabolic alkalosis
   C. Compensated metabolic acidosis
   D. Compensated metabolic alkalosis

6. If a person hyperventilates for a given time period, which of the following will probably develop?
   A. Metabolic acidosis
   B. Metabolic alkalosis
   C. Respiratory acidosis
   D. Respiratory alkalosis

7. What happens when lactic acid dissociates in the blood?
   A. H+ is added to blood.
   B. pH is lowered.
   C. Acidosis results.
   D. All of the above

8. Which of the following is *true* of metabolic alkalosis?
   A. It occurs in the case of prolonged vomiting.
   B. It results when the bicarbonate ion is present in excess.
   C. Therapy includes intravenous administration of normal saline.
   D. All of the above

9. Which of the following is a characteristic of a buffer system in the body?
   A. It prevents drastic changes from occurring in body pH.
   B. It picks up both hydrogen and hydroxide ions.
   C. It is exemplified by the bicarbonate-carbonic acid system
   D. All of the above
10. In the presence of a strong acid, which of the following is *true*?
    A. Sodium bicarbonate will react to produce carbonic acid.
    B. Sodium bicarbonate will react to produce more sodium bicarbonate.
    C. Carbonic acid will react to produce sodium bicarbonate.
    D. Carbonic acid will react to form more carbonic acid.

Matching

Select the most appropriate answer from column B for each item in column A. There is only one correct answer for each item.

Column A
_____ 11. pH lower than 7.0
_____ 12. pH higher than 7.0
_____ 13. Buffers
_____ 14. Decrease in respirations
_____ 15. Increase in respirations
_____ 16. Metabolic acidosis
_____ 17. Metabolic alkalosis
_____ 18. Lactic acid
_____ 19. Kidney
_____ 20. Uncompensated metabolic acidosis

Column B
A. Bicarbonate deficit
B. Bicarbonate excess
C. Alkaline solution
D. "Fixed" acid
E. Respiratory acidosis
F. Respiratory alkalosis
G. Acidic solution
H. Lower than normal ratio of sodium bicarbonate to carbonic acid
I. Prevent sharp pH changes
J. Most effective regulators of body pH

CHAPTER 19 The Reproductive Systems

The reproductive system consists of those organs that participate in perpetuating the species. It is a unique body system in that its organs differ between the two sexes and yet they work toward the same goal: creating a new being. Of interest also is the fact that this system is the only one not necessary to the survival of the individual, and yet survival of the species depends on its proper functioning. The male reproductive system is divided into the external genitals, the testes, the duct system, and the accessory glands. The testes, or gonads, are considered essential organs because they produce the sex cells, sperm, that join with the female sex cells, ova, to form a new human being. They also secrete the male sex hormone, testosterone, which is responsible for the physical transformation of a boy into a man.

Sperm are formed in the testes by the seminiferous tubules. From there they enter a long narrow duct, the epididymis. They continue onward through the vas deferens into the ejaculatory duct, down the urethra, and out of the body. Throughout this journey, various glands secrete substances that add motility to the sperm and create a chemical environment that is conducive to reproduction.

The female reproductive system is truly extraordinary and diverse. It produces ova, receives the penis and sperm during intercourse, serves as the site of conception, houses and feeds the embryo during prenatal development, and nourishes the infant after birth.

Because of its diversity, the physiology of the female is generally considered to be more complex than that of the male. Much of the activity of this system revolves around the menstrual cycle and the monthly preparation that the female undergoes for a possible pregnancy.

The organs of the female system are divided into essential organs and accessory organs of reproduction. The essential organs of the female are the ovaries. Just as with the male, the essential organs of the female are referred to as the gonads. The gonads of both sexes produce the sex cells. In the male, the gonads produce the sperm and in the female they produce the ova. The gonads are also responsible for producing the hormones in each sex necessary for the appearance of the secondary sex characteristics.

The menstrual cycle of the female typically covers a period of 28 days. Each cycle consists of three phases: the menstrual period, the postmenstrual phase, and the premenstrual phase. Changes in the blood levels of the hormones that are responsible for the menstrual cycle also cause physical and emotional changes in the female. A knowledge of these phenomena and this system, in both the male and the female, are necessary to complete your understanding of the reproductive system.

TOPICS FOR REVIEW

Before progressing to Chapter 20, you should familiarize yourself with the structure and function of the organs of the male and female reproductive systems. Your review should include emphasis on the gross and microscopic structure of the testes and the production of sperm and testosterone. Your study should continue by tracing the pathway of a sperm cell from formation to expulsion from the body.

You should then familiarize yourself with the structure and function of the organs of the female reproductive system. Your review should include emphasis on the development of a mature ovum from ovarian follicles and should also concentrate on the phases and occurrences in a typical 28-day menstrual cycle.

MALE REPRODUCTIVE SYSTEM STRUCTURAL PLAN

Match the term on the left with the proper selection on the right.

Group A

_____ 1. Testes
_____ 2. Spermatozoa
_____ 3. Ova
_____ 4. Penis
_____ 5. Zygote

A. Fertilized ovum
B. Accessory organ
C. Male sex cell
D. Gonads
E. Gamete

Group B

_____ 6. Testes
_____ 7. Bulbourethral
_____ 8. Asexual
_____ 9. External genitalia
_____ 10. Prostate

A. Cowper's gland
B. Scrotum
C. Essential organ
D. Single parent
E. Accessory organ

▶ *If you have had difficulty with this section, review pages 453-454.*

TESTES

Circle the correct answer.

11. The testes are surrounded by a tough membrane called the:
    A. Ductus deferens
    B. Tunica albuginea
    C. Septum
    D. Seminiferous membrane

12. The _____ lie near the septa that separate the lobules.
    A. Ductus deferens
    B. Sperm
    C. Interstitial cells
    D. Nerves

13. Sperm are found in the walls of the:
    A. Seminiferous tubule
    B. Interstitial cells
    C. Septum
    D. Blood vessels
14. An undescended testicle is called a(n):
    A. Orchidalgia
    B. Orchidorrhaphy
    C. Orchichorea
    D. Cryptorchidism
15. The structure(s) that produce(s) testosterone is(are) the:
    A. Seminiferous tubules
    B. Prostate gland
    C. Bulbourethral gland
    D. Pituitary gland
    E. Interstitial cells
16. The part of the sperm that contains genetic information that will be inherited is the:
    A. Tail
    B. Neck
    C. Middle piece
    D. Head
    E. Acrosome
17. Which one of the following is *not* a function of testosterone?
    A. It causes a deepening of the voice.
    B. It promotes the development of the male accessory glands.
    C. It has a stimulatory effect on protein catabolism.
    D. It causes greater muscular development and strength.
18. Sperm production is called:
    A. Spermatogonia
    B. Spermatids
    C. Spermatogenesis
    D. Spermatocyte
19. The section of the sperm that contains enzymes that enable it to break down the covering of the ovum and permit entry should contact occur is the:
    A. Acrosome
    B. Midpiece
    C. Tail
    D. Stem
20. Descent of the testes usually occurs about:
    A. Two months after birth
    B. Two months before birth
    C. Two months after conception
    D. Two years after birth
    E. None of the above

Fill in the blanks.

The (21) _____ are the gonads of the male. From puberty on, the seminiferous tubules are continuously forming (22) _____. Any of these cells may join with the female sex cell, the (23) _____, to become a new human being.

Another function of the testes is to secrete the male hormone (24) _____, which transforms a boy to a man. This hormone is secreted by the (25) _____ _____ of the testes. A good way to remember testosterone's functions is to think of it as "the (26) _____ hormone" and "the (27) _____ hormone."

 If you have had difficulty with this section, review pages 455-459.

REPRODUCTIVE DUCTS
ACCESSORY OR SUPPORTIVE SEX GLANDS
EXTERNAL GENITALIA

Choose the correct term and write the letter in the space next to the appropriate definition below.

A. Epididymis
B. Vas deferens
C. Ejaculatory duct
D. Prepuce
E. Seminal vesicles

F. Prostate gland
G. Cowper's gland
H. Prostatectomy
I. Semen
J. Scrotum

_____ 28. Continuation of ducts that start in epididymis
_____ 29. Procedure performed for benign prostatic hypertrophy
_____ 30. Also known as "bulbourethral"
_____ 31. Narrow tube that lies along the top of and behind the testes
_____ 32. Doughnut-shaped gland beneath bladder
_____ 33. Continuation of vas deferens
_____ 34. Mixture of sperm and secretions of accessory sex glands
_____ 35. Contributes 60% of the seminal fluid volume
_____ 36. Removed during circumcision
_____ 37. External genitalia

If you have had difficulty with this section, review pages 460-462.

FEMALE REPRODUCTIVE SYSTEM STRUCTURAL PLAN

Match the term on the left with the proper selection on the right.

———— 38. Ovaries   A. Genitals
———— 39. Vagina   B. Accessory sex gland
———— 40. Bartholin   C. Accessory duct
———— 41. Vulva   D. Gonads
———— 42. Ova   E. Sex cells

Select the correct term from the options given and write the letter in the answer blank.

A. External structure   B. Internal structure

———— 43. Mons pubis
———— 44. Vagina
———— 45. Labia majora
———— 46. Uterine tubes
———— 47. Vestibule
———— 48. Clitoris
———— 49. Labia minora
———— 50. Ovaries

 If you have had difficulty with this section, review pages 462-467.

OVARIES

Fill in the blanks.

The ovaries are the (51) ————————— of the female. They have two main functions. The first is the production of the female sex cell. This process is called (52) —————————. The specialized type of cell division that occurs during sexual cell reproduction is known as (53) —————————. The ovum is the body's largest cell and has (54) ————————— the number of chromosomes found in other body cells. At the time of (55) —————————, the sex cells from both parents fuse and (56) ————————— chromosomes are united.

The second major function of the ovaries is to secrete the sex hormones (57) ————————— and (58) —————————. Estrogen is the sex hormone that causes the development and maintenance of the female (59) ————————— ————————— —————————. Progesterone acts with estrogen to help initiate the (60)

————————— ————————— in girls entering (61) —————————.

 If you have had difficulty with this section, review pages 462-465.

FEMALE REPRODUCTIVE DUCTS

Select the correct term from the options given and write the letter in the answer blank.

      A. Uterine tubes   B. Uterus   C. Vagina

_____ 62. Ectopic pregnancy
_____ 63. Lining known as endometrium
_____ 64. Terminal end of birth canal
_____ 65. Site of menstruation
_____ 66. Approximately 4 inches in length
_____ 67. Consists of body, fundus, and cervix
_____ 68. Site of fertilization
_____ 69. Also known as "oviduct"
_____ 70. Entrance way for sperm
_____ 71. Total hysterectomy

 If you have had difficulty with this section, review pages 465-471.

ACCESSORY OR SUPPORTIVE SEX GLANDS EXTERNAL GENITALS OF THE FEMALE

Match the term on the left with the proper selection on the right.

Group A

_____ 72. Bartholin's gland   A. Colored area around nipple
_____ 73. Breasts   B. Grape-like clusters of milk-secreting cells
_____ 74. Alveoli   C. Drain alveoli
_____ 75. Lactiferous ducts   D. Secretes lubricating fluid
_____ 76. Areola   E. Primarily fat tissue

Group B

_____ 77. Mons pubis   A. "Large lips"
_____ 78. Labia majora   B. Area between labia minora
_____ 79. Clitoris   C. Surgical procedure
_____ 80. Vestibule   D. Composed of erectile tissue
_____ 81. Episiotomy   E. Pad of fat over the symphysis pubis

If you have had difficulty with this section, review pages 466-468.

MENSTRUAL CYCLE

If the statement is true, write "T" in the answer blank. If the statement is false, correct the statement by circling the incorrect term and writing the correct term in the answer blank.

_____ 82. "Climacteric" is the scientific name for the beginning of the menses.
_____ 83. As a general rule, several ovum mature each month during the 30 to 40 years that a woman has menstrual periods.

_____ 84. Ovulation occurs 28 days before the next menstrual period begins.

_____ 85. The first day of ovulation is considered the first day of the cycle.

_____ 86. A woman's fertile period lasts only a few days out of each month.

_____ 87. The control of the menstrual cycle lies in the posterior pituitary gland.

Write the letter of the correct hormone in the blank next to the appropriate description.

A. FSH   B. LH

_____ 88. Ovulating hormone

_____ 89. Secreted during the first days of menstrual cycle

_____ 90. Secreted after the estrogen level of blood increases

_____ 91. Causes final maturation of the follicle and ovum

_____ 92. Birth control pills suppress this hormone

 If you have had difficulty with this section, review pages 468-471.

APPLYING WHAT YOU KNOW

93. Mr. Belinki is going into the hospital for the surgical removal of his testes. As a result of this surgery, will Mr. Belinki be impotent? Why or why not?

_____

_____

_____

94. When baby Ross was born, the pediatrician discovered that his left testicle had not descended into the scrotum. If this situation is not corrected soon, might baby Ross be sterile or impotent? Why or why not?

_____

_____

_____

95. Ms. Gaynes contracted gonorrhea. By the time she made an appointment to see her doctor, it had spread to her abdominal organs. How is this possible when gonorrhea is a disease of the reproductive system?

_____

_____

_____

_____

96. Mrs. Harlan was having a bilateral oophorectomy. Is this a sterilization procedure? Will she experience menopause?

_____

_____

_____

97. Delceta had a total hysterectomy. Will she experience menopause?

_____

_____

_____

98. WORD FIND

Can you find 18 terms from this chapter? Words may be spelled top to bottom, bottom to top, right to left, left to right, or diagonally.

```
M  K  O  V  I  D  U  C  T  S  E  D  H  G
S  E  I  R  A  V  O  I  F  U  T  G  L  L
I  N  H  Z  H  M  P  M  K  O  H  I  C  W
D  D  V  A  S  D  E  F  E  R  E  N  S  H
I  O  A  C  C  I  P  J  V  E  H  Y  D  S
H  M  G  R  R  B  M  N  X  F  G  Y  I  O
C  E  I  O  O  E  Z  Y  T  I  C  S  T  E
R  T  N  S  T  P  S  D  D  N  O  V  A  D
O  R  A  O  U  W  E  B  A  I  J  S  M  Z
T  I  C  M  M  E  Y  N  E  M  D  L  R  V
P  U  A  E  U  D  G  M  I  E  H  I  E  H
Y  M  O  T  C  E  T  A  T  S  O  R  P  B
R  P  E  E  R  M  N  E  G  O  R  T  S  E
C  O  W  P  E  R  S  I  N  X  K  E  A  P
```

Acrosome   Meiosis   Scrotum
Cowpers   Ovaries   Seminiferous
Cryptorchidism Oviducts   Sperm
Endometrium   Penis   Spermatids
Epididymis   Pregnancy   Vagina
Estrogen   Prostatectomy   Vas deferens

DID YOU KNOW?

The testes produce approximately 50 million sperm per day. Every 2 to 3 months, every fertile man produces enough sperm cells to populate the entire earth.

REPRODUCTIVE SYSTEM

Fill in the crossword puzzle.

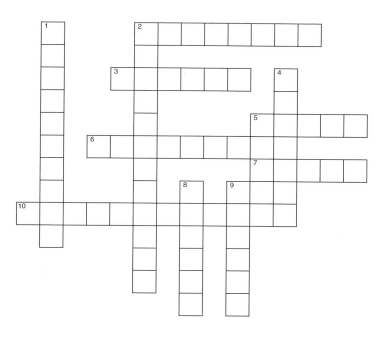

Across

2. Female erectile tissue
3. Colored area around the nipple
5. Male reproductive fluid
6. Sex cells
7. External genitalia
10. Male sex hormone

Down

1. Failure to have a menstrual period
2. Surgical removal of the foreskin
4. Foreskin
8. Menstrual period
9. Essential organs of reproduction

CHECK YOUR KNOWLEDGE
Multiple Choice

Circle the correct answer.

1. What is the membrane that may cover the vaginal opening of the female called?
   A. Hymen
   B. Mons pubis
   C. Labia
   D. Clitoris

2. Which of the following statements about the menstrual cycle is *true*?
   A. Estrogen levels are lowest at the time of ovulation.
   B. Progesterone levels are highest at the time of ovulation.
   C. FSH levels are highest during the proliferation phase.
   D. None of the above

3. Semen could contain which of the following?
   A. Sperm cells
   B. Secretion from the prostate
   C. Secretions from the seminal vesicles
   D. All of the above

4. What is the failure of the testes to descend into the scrotum before birth called?
   A. Cryptococcoses
   B. Coccidioidomycosis
   C. Cryptorchidism
   D. Cholelithiasis

5. Which of the following is *not* an accessory organ of the female reproductive system?
   A. Breast
   B. Bartholin's glands
   C. Ovary
   D. All of the above are accessory organs

6. Which of the following structures can be referred to as male gonads?
   A. Testes
   B. Epididymis
   C. Vas deferens
   D. All of the above

7. Sperm cells are suspended outside of the body cavity so as to do which of the following?
   A. Protect them from trauma
   B. Keep them at a cooler temperature
   C. Keep them supplied with a greater number of blood vessels
   D. Protect them from infection

8. What is the removal of the foreskin from the glans penis called?
   A. Vasectomy
   B. Sterilization
   C. Circumcision
   D. Ligation

9. What is the colored area around the nipple of the breast called?
   A. Areola
   B. Lactiferous duct
   C. Alveoli
   D. None of the above
10. Which of the following is *true* about the postmenstrual phase of the menstrual cycle?
    A. The endometrium is being repaired.
    B. Luteinizing hormone is secreted.
    C. Progesterone is being secreted.
    D. All of the above

Completion

Complete the following statements using the terms listed below:

A. Clitoris	G. Hysterectomy
B. Endometrium	H. Prostate
C. Ectopic	I. FSH (follicle-stimulating hormone)
D. Corpus luteum	J. Ovulation
E. Menses	K. Scrotum
F. Epididymis	L. Testosterone

11. A pregnancy resulting from the implantation of a fertilized ovum in any location other than the uterus is called _____.
12. Interstitial cells of the testes function to produce _____.
13. The doughnut-shaped accessory organ or gland that surrounds the male urethra is called the _____.
14. Surgical removal of the uterus is called _____.
15. The _____ houses sperm cells as they mature and develop their ability to swim.
16. The skin-covered external pouch that contains the testes is called the _____.
17. The lining of the uterus is called _____.
18. The hormone progesterone is secreted by a structure called the _____.
19. Fertilization of an egg by a sperm can only occur around the time of _____.
20. From about the first to the seventh day of the menstrual cycle, the anterior pituitary gland secretes _____.

Male Reproductive Organs

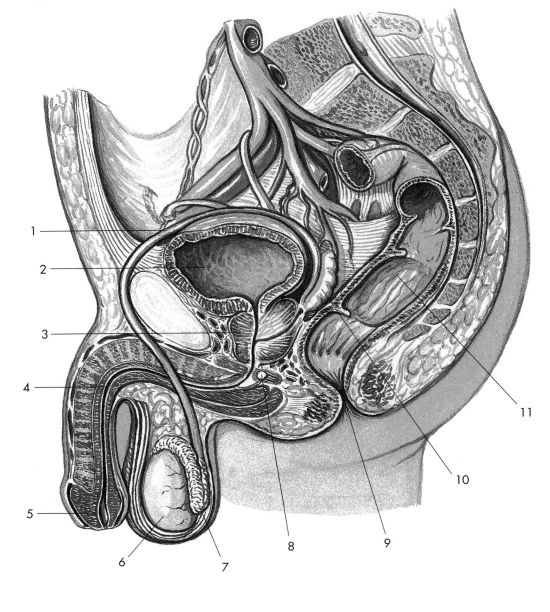

1. _____

2. _____

3. _____

4. _____

5. _____

6. _____

7. _____

8. _____

9. _____

10. _____

11. _____

Tubules of Testis and Epididymis

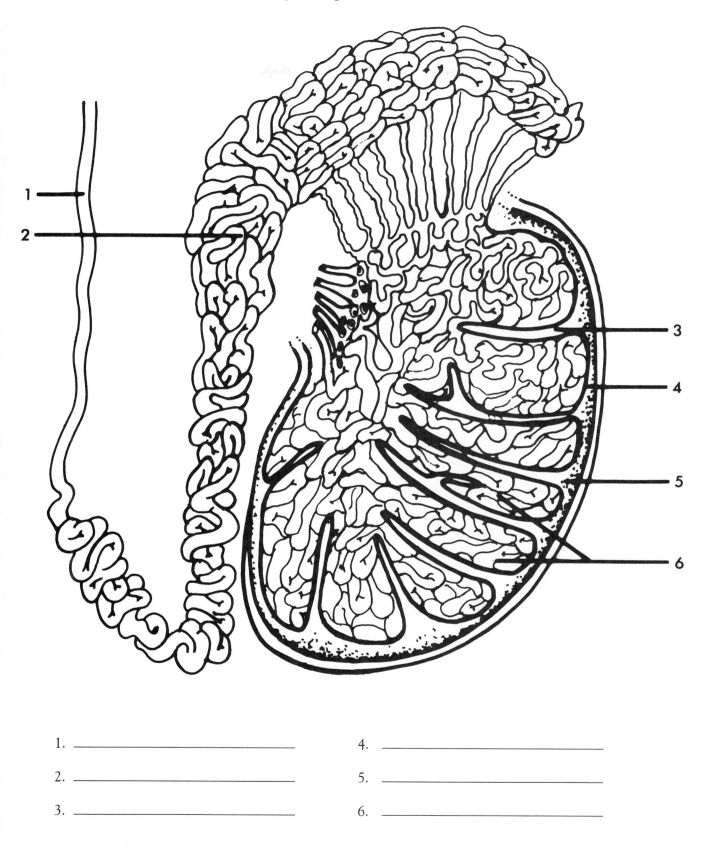

1. _____ 4. _____

2. _____ 5. _____

3. _____ 6. _____

Vulva

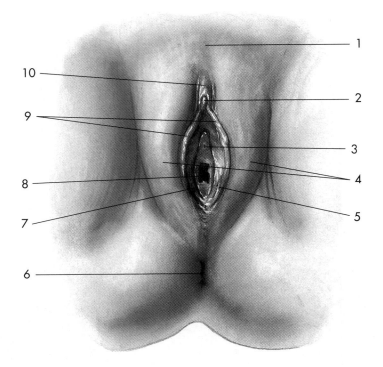

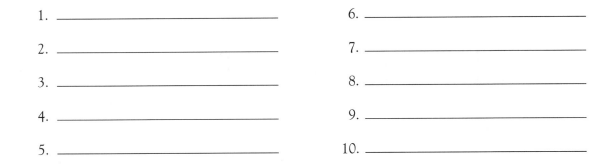

1. _____

2. _____

3. _____

4. _____

5. _____

6. _____

7. _____

8. _____

9. _____

10. _____

Breast

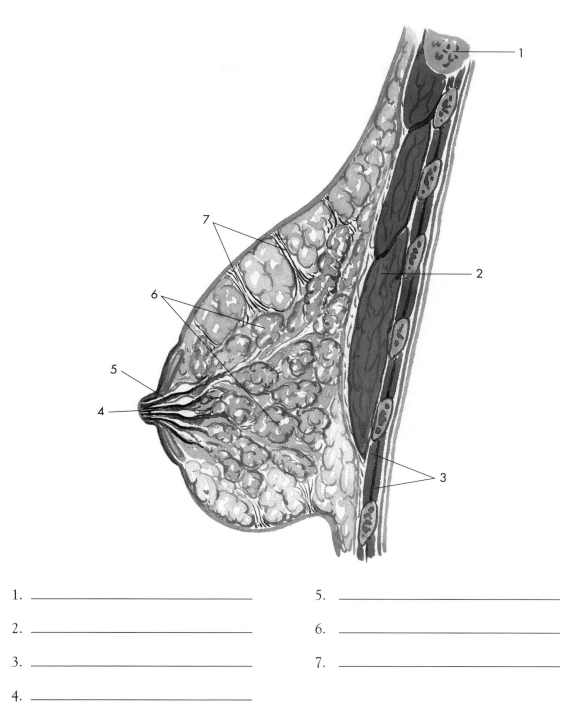

1. _____   5. _____

2. _____   6. _____

3. _____   7. _____

4. _____

Female Pelvis

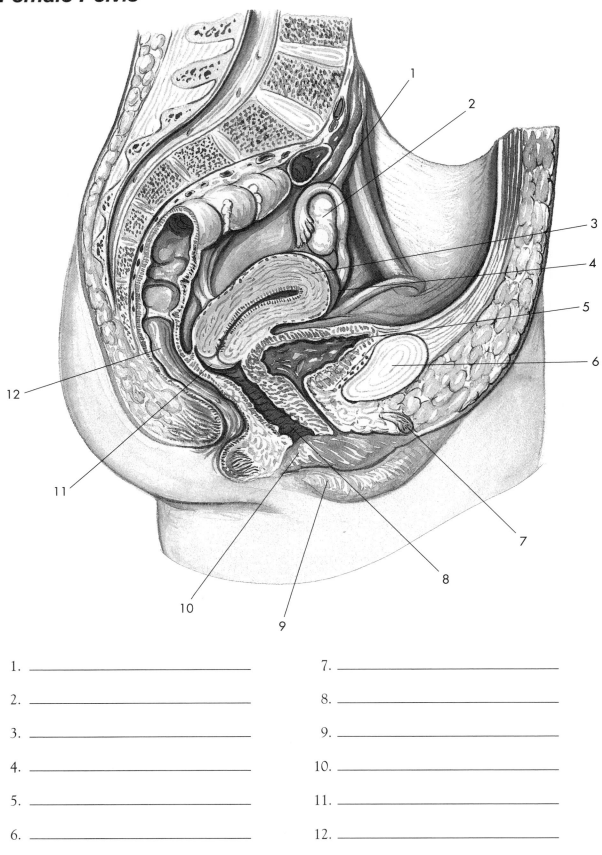

1. _____
2. _____
3. _____
4. _____
5. _____
6. _____

7. _____
8. _____
9. _____
10. _____
11. _____
12. _____

Uterus and Adjacent Structures

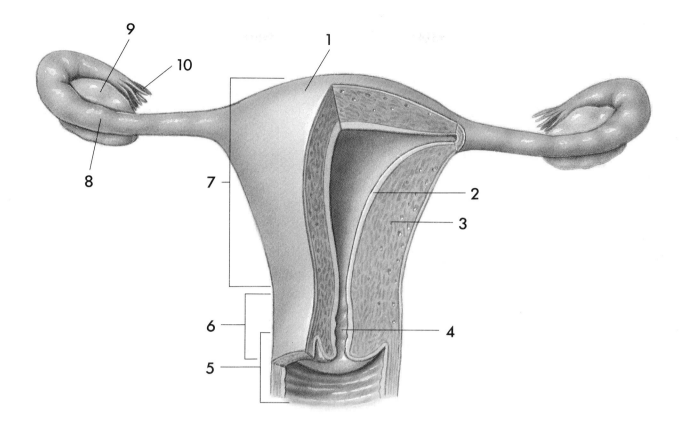

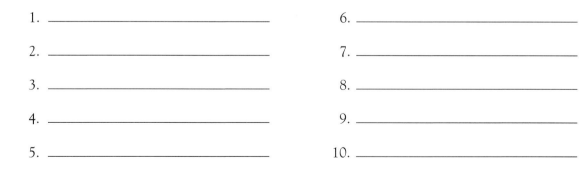

1. _____
2. _____
3. _____
4. _____
5. _____

6. _____
7. _____
8. _____
9. _____
10. _____

CHAPTER 20 Growth and Development

Millions of fragile microscopic sperm swim against numerous obstacles to reach the ova and create a new life. At birth, the newborn will fill his lungs with air and cry lustily, signaling to the world that he is ready to begin the cycle of life. This cycle will be marked by ongoing changes, periodic physical growth, and continuous development.

This chapter reviews the more significant events that occur in the normal growth and development of an individual from conception to death. Realizing that each individual is unique, we nonetheless can discover, amid all the complexities of humanity, some constants that are understandable and predictable.

A knowledge of human growth and development is essential in understanding the commonalties that influence individuals as they pass through the cycle of life.

TOPICS FOR REVIEW

Your review of this chapter should include an understanding of the concept of development as a biological process. You should familiarize yourself with the major developmental changes from conception through older adulthood. Your study should conclude with a review of the effects of aging on the body systems.

PRENATAL PERIOD

Fill in the blanks.

The prenatal stage of development begins at the time of (1) _____ and continues until (2) _____. The science of the development of an individual before birth is called (3) _____.

Fertilization takes place in the outer third of the (4) _____. The fertilized ovum, or (5) _____, begins to divide and in approximately 3 days forms a solid mass called a (6) _____. By the time it enters the uterus, it is a hollow ball of cells called a (7) _____.

As it continues to develop, it forms a structure with two cavities. The (8) _____ _____ will become a fluid-filled sac for the embryo. The (9) _____ will develop into an important fetal membrane in the (10) _____.

Choose the correct term and write the letter in the space next to the appropriate definition below.

A. Laparoscope
B. Gestation
C. Antenatal
D. Histogenesis
E. Quickening

F. Endoderm
G. In vitro
H. Parturition
I. Embryonic phase
J. Ultrasonogram

_____ 11. "Within a glass"
_____ 12. Inside germ layer
_____ 13. Before birth
_____ 14. Length of pregnancy
_____ 15. Fiberoptic viewing instrument
_____ 16. Process of birth
_____ 17. First fetal movement
_____ 18. Study of how the primary germ layers develop into many different kinds of tissues
_____ 19. Fertilization until the end of the eighth week of gestation
_____ 20. Monitors the progress of the developing fetus

▶ *If you have had difficulty with this section, review pages 482-491.*

POSTNATAL PERIOD

Circle the correct answer.

21. During the postnatal period:
    A. The head becomes proportionately smaller
    B. Thoracic and abdominal contours change from round to elliptical
    C. The legs become proportionately longer
    D. The trunk becomes proportionately shorter
    E. All of the above

22. The period of infancy starts at birth and lasts about:
    A. 4 weeks
    B. 4 months
    C. 10 weeks
    D. 12 months
    E. 18 months

23. The lumbar curvature of the spine appears _____ months after birth.
    A. 1-10
    B. 5-8
    C. 8-12
    D. 11-15
    E. 12-18

24. During the first 4 months after birth, the birth weight will:
    A. Double
    B. Triple
    C. Quadruple
    D. None of the above

25. At the end of the first year, the weight of the baby will have:
    A. Doubled
    B. Tripled
    C. Quadrupled
    D. None of the above

26. The infant is capable of following a moving object with its eyes at the age of:
    A. 2 days
    B. 2 weeks
    C. 2 months
    D. 4 months
    E. 10 months

27. The infant can lift its head and raise its chest at the age of:
    A. 2 months
    B. 3 months
    C. 4 months
    D. 10 months

28. The infant can crawl at the age of:
    A. 2 months
    B. 3 months
    C. 4 months
    D. 10 months
    E. 12 months

29. The infant can stand alone at the age of:
    A. 2 months
    B. 3 months
    C. 4 months
    D. 10 months
    E. 12 months
30. The permanent teeth, with the exception of the third molar, have all erupted by age _____ years.
    A. 6
    B. 8
    C. 12
    D. 14
    E. None of the above
31. Puberty starts at age _____ years in boys.
    A. 10-13
    B. 12-14
    C. 14-16
    D. None of the above
32. Most girls begin breast development at about age:
    A. 8
    B. 9
    C. 10
    D. 11
    E. 12
33. The growth spurt is generally complete by age _____ in males.
    A. 14
    B. 15
    C. 16
    D. 18
34. An average age at which girls begin to menstruate is _____ years.
    A. 10-12
    B. 11-12
    C. 12-13
    D. 13-14
    E. 14-15
35. The first sign of puberty in boys is:
    A. Facial hair
    B. Increased muscle mass
    C. Pubic hair
    D. Deepening of the voice
    E. Increased testicular enlargement

Write the letter of the correct word in the blank next to the appropriate definition.

A. Neonatology
B. Neonatal
C. Adolescence
D. Deciduous
E. Puberty

F. Postnatal
G. Infancy
H. Childhood
I. Senescence

_____ 36. Begins at birth and lasts until death
_____ 37. Concerned with the diagnosis and treatment of disorders of the newborn
_____ 38. Teenage years
_____ 39. From the end of infancy to puberty
_____ 40. Baby teeth
_____ 41. First 4 weeks of infancy
_____ 42. Secondary sexual characteristics occur
_____ 43. Begins at birth and lasts about 18 months
_____ 44. Old age

 If you have had difficulty with this section, review pages 491-495.

EFFECTS OF AGING

Fill in the blanks.

45. Old bones develop indistinct and shaggy margins with spurs, a process called _____.
46. A degenerative joint disease common in the aged is _____.
47. The number of _____ units in the kidney decreases by almost 50% between the ages of 30 and 75.
48. During old age, respiratory efficiency decreases, and a condition known as _____ _____ results.
49. Fatty deposits accumulate in blood vessels as we age, and the result is _____ which narrows the passageway for the flow of blood.
50. Hardening of the arteries or _____ occurs during the aging process.
51. Another term for high blood pressure is _____.
52. Hardening of the lens is _____.
53. If the lens becomes cloudy and impairs vision, it is called a _____.
54. _____ causes an increase in the pressure within the eyeball and may result in blindness.

 If you have had difficulty with this section, review pages 495-497.

UNSCRAMBLE THE WORDS

55. ANNFCYI

56. NAALTTSOP

57. OGSSNEGRAONEI

58. GTEYZO

59. HDOOLHCID

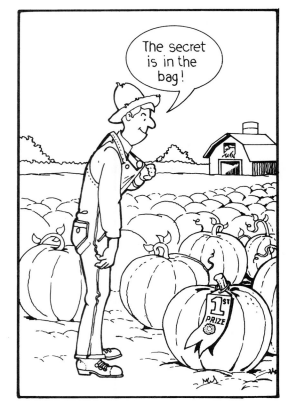

Take the circled letters, unscramble them, and fill in the statement.

The secret to Farmer Brown's prize pumpkin crop.

60.

APPLYING WHAT YOU KNOW

61. Heather's mother told the pediatrician during Heather's 1-year visit that Heather had tripled her birth weight, was crawling actively, and could stand alone. Is Heather's development normal, retarded, or advanced?

_____

62. Clarke is 70 years old. She has always enjoyed food and has had a hearty appetite. Lately, however, she has complained that food "just doesn't taste as good anymore." What might be a possible explanation?

_____

_____

63. Mr. Altman, age 68, has noticed hearing problems, but only under certain circumstances. He has difficulty with certain tones, especially high or low tones, but has no problem with everyday conversation. What might be a possible explanation?

_____

_____

64. WORD FIND

Can you find 14 terms from this chapter? Words may be spelled top to bottom, bottom to top, right to left, left to right, or diagonally.

```
F  T  P  N  O  I  T  A  T  S  E  G  K  F  U
Z  E  P  O  C  S  O  R  A  P  A  L  H  E  A
E  O  R  I  L  T  O  H  H  O  C  J  V  J  T
C  M  V  T  N  T  I  M  L  N  L  Z  P  U  O
M  A  B  I  I  F  R  M  R  E  D  O  T  C  E
H  Q  C  R  D  L  A  M  E  S  O  D  E  R  M
N  N  M  U  Y  U  I  N  M  F  O  W  G  O  P
K  N  V  T  C  O  Z  C  H  H  F  R  C  N
H  G  Y  R  K  L  T  A  Y  D  U  C  V  P
L  A  T  A  N  T  S  O  P  T  L  U  N  Q  G
Q  N  K  P  Y  Y  S  W  G  A  I  K  E  M  T
U  G  P  Q  N  H  O  Y  X  Y  H  O  Z  B  N
I  Y  T  R  E  B  U  P  L  A  C  E  N  T  A
```

Childhood   Infancy   Parturition
Ectoderm   Laparoscope   Placenta
Embryology   Mesoderm   Postnatal
Fertilization Morula   Puberty
Gestation   Oviduct

DID YOU KNOW?

Brain cells do not regenerate. One beer permanently destroys 10,000 cells.

GROWTH/DEVELOPMENT

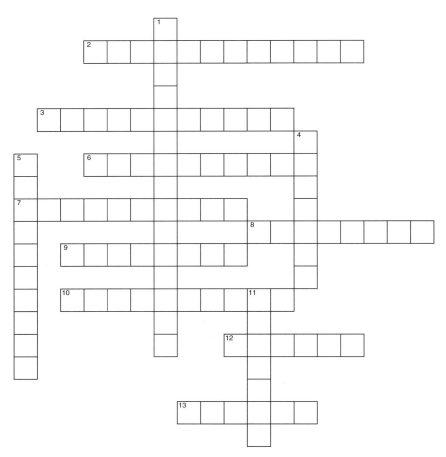

Across

2. Study of how germ layers develop into tissues
3. Process of birth
6. Name of zygote after implantation
7. Science of the development of the individual before birth
8. Eye disease marked by increased pressure in the eyeball
9. Cloudy lens
10. Old age
12. Name of zygote after 3 days
13. Fertilized ovum

Down

1. Fatty deposit buildup on walls of arteries
4. First 4 weeks of infancy
5. Hardening of the lens
11. Will develop into a fetal membrane in the placenta

CHECK YOUR KNOWLEDGE

Multiple Choice

Circle the correct answer.

1. When the human embryo is a hollow ball of cells consisting of an outer cell layer and an inner cell mass, what is it called?
   A. Morula
   B. Chorion
   C. Blastocyst
   D. Zygote

2. Degenerative changes in the urinary system that accompany old age include which of the following?
   A. Decreased capacity of bladder and the inability to empty or void completely
   B. Decrease in the number of nephrons
   C. Less blood flow through the kidneys
   D. All of the above

3. The frontal and maxillary sinuses of the facial region acquire permanent placement or develop fully when the individual is in a stage of development known as:
   A. Infancy
   B. Childhood
   C. Adolescence
   D. Adulthood

4. The first 4 weeks of human life after birth are referred to as which of the following?
   A. Neonatal
   B. Infancy
   C. Prenatal
   D. Embryonic

5. Any hardening of the arteries is referred to as which of the following?
   A. Angioma
   B. Atherosclerosis
   C. Angina
   D. Arteriosclerosis

6. Which of the following is characteristic of the disorder called presbyopia?
   A. It is very characteristic of old age.
   B. It causes farsightedness in some individuals.
   C. It is characterized by a lens in the eye becoming hard and losing its elasticity.
   D. All of the above

7. Which of the following events is *not* characteristic of infancy?
   A. One spinal curvature is present
   B. The head accounts for approximately one fourth of total body height
   C. Quickening apparent
   D. 50% increase in body length

8. Which of the following events is *not* characteristic of adolescence?
   A. Bone closure
   B. Development of secondary sexual characteristics
   C. Very rapid growth
   D. All of the above events are characteristic of adolescence.

9. Which of the following events is *not* characteristic of the prenatal period of development?
   A. Blastocyst is formed.
   B. Histogenesis occurs.
   C. Bone closure occurs.
   D. Amniotic cavity is formed.
10. Which of the following structures is derived from ectoderm?
   A. Lining of lungs
   B. Brain
   C. Kidneys
   D. All of the above

Matching

Select the most appropriate answer from column B for each item in column A. There is only one correct answer for each item.

Column A
_____ 11. Arteriosclerosis
_____ 12. Atherosclerosis
_____ 13. Parturition
_____ 14. Cataract
_____ 15. Adolescence
_____ 16. Amniotic sac
_____ 17. Glaucoma
_____ 18. Senescence
_____ 19. Hypertension
_____ 20. Placenta

Column B
A. High blood pressure
B. Chorion
C. Birth
D. "Bag of waters"
E. Hardening of arteries
F. Degeneration
G. Fat accumulation in arteries
H. Secondary sexual characteristics
I. Clouding of eye lens
J. High eye pressure

Fertilization and Implantation

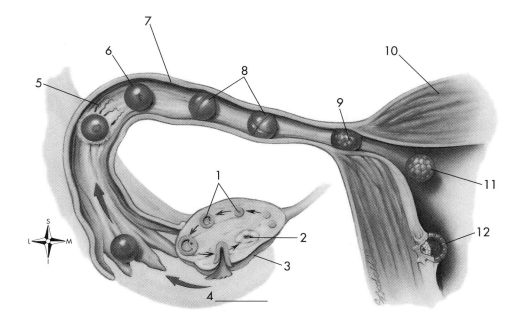

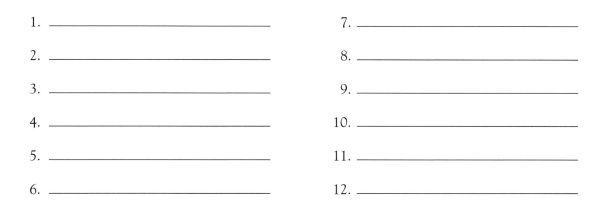

1. _____   7. _____

2. _____   8. _____

3. _____   9. _____

4. _____   10. _____

5. _____   11. _____

6. _____   12. _____

Answer Key

CHAPTER 1
AN INTRODUCTION TO THE STRUCTURE AND FUNCTION OF THE BODY

Matching

1. D, p. 2
2. E, p. 2
3. A, p. 2
4. C, p. 2
5. B, p. 2

Matching

6. C, p. 2
7. A, p. 2
8. E, p. 2
9. D, p. 2
10. B, p. 2

Crossword puzzle

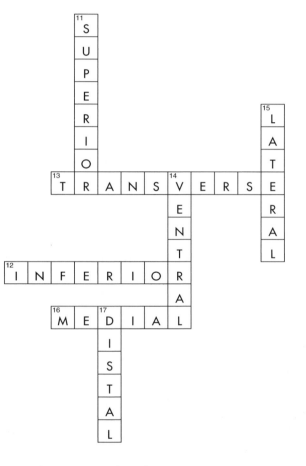

Did you notice that the answers were arranged as they appear on the human body?

Circle the correct answer

18. Inferior, p. 4
19. Anterior, p. 4
20. Lateral, p. 4
21. Proximal, p. 4
22. Superficial, p. 4
23. Equal, p. 6
24. Anterior and posterior, p. 6
25. Upper and lower, p. 6
26. Frontal, p. 6

Select the correct term

27. A, p. 6
28. B, p. 7
29. A, p. 7
30. A, p. 7
31. A, p. 7
32. B, p. 7
33. A, p. 7

Circle the one that does *not* belong

34. Extremities (all others are part of the axial portions)
35. Cephalic (all others are part of the arm)
36. Plantar (all others are part of the face)
37. Carpal (all others are part of the leg or foot)
38. Tarsal (all others are part of the skull)

Fill in the blanks

39. Survival, p. 12
40. Internal environment, p. 12
41. Feedback loop, p. 12
42. Negative, positive, p. 12
43. Stabilize, p. 12
44. Stimulatory, p. 12
45. Developmental processes, p. 14
46. Aging processes, p. 14

Applying what you know

47. ① on diagram
48. ② on diagram
49. ③ on diagram

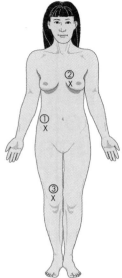

50. WORD FIND

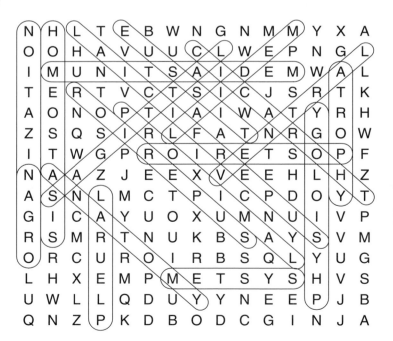

Check your knowledge

MULTIPLE CHOICE

1. A, p. 12
2. D, p. 7
3. B, p. 8
4. D, p. 6
5. A, p. 1
6. C, p. 6
7. C, p. 2
8. A, p. 6
9. C, p. 8
10. B, p. 7
11. D, p. 8
12. B, p. 8
13. C, p. 2
14. D, p. 6
15. D, p. 4
16. A, p. 2
17. D, p. 10
18. A, p. 8
19. A, p. 10
20. C, p. 4

MATCHING

21. F, p. 5
22. B, p. 11
23. J, p. 6
24. G, p. 1
25. H, p. 4
26. C, p. 8
27. D, p. 10
28. I, p. 4
29. A, p. 6
30. E, p. 2

DORSAL AND VENTRAL BODY CAVITIES

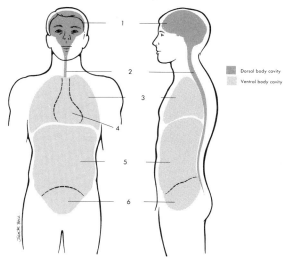

1. Cranial cavity
2. Spinal cavity
3. Thoracic cavity
4. Mediastinum
5. Abdominal cavity
6. Pelvic cavity

DIRECTIONS AND PLANES OF THE BODY

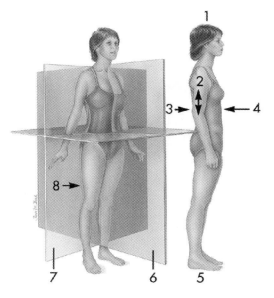

1. Superior
2. Proximal
3. Posterior (dorsal)
4. Anterior (ventral)
5. Inferior
6. Sagittal plane
7. Frontal plane
8. Lateral

Answer Key   273

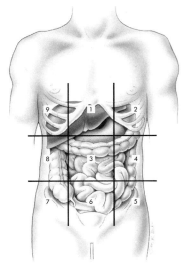

1. Epigastric region
2. Left hypochondriac region
3. Umbilical region
4. Left lumbar region
5. Left iliac (inguinal) region
6. Hypogastric region
7. Right iliac (inguinal) region
8. Right lumbar region
9. Right hypochondriac region

CHAPTER 2
CELLS AND TISSUES

Matching

1. C, p. 22
2. E, p. 22
3. A, p. 22
4. B, p. 27
5. D, p. 26
6. D, p. 25
7. E, p. 25
8. A, p. 25
9. B, p. 25
10. C, p. 26

Fill in the blanks

11. Organelles, p. 22
12. Tissue typing, p. 22
13. Cilia, p. 25
14. Aerobic or cellular respiration, p. 26
15. Ribosomes, p. 25
16. Mitochondria, p. 26
17. Lysosomes, p. 26
18. Golgi apparatus, p. 26
19. Centrioles, p. 26
20. Chromatin granules, p. 27

Circle the correct answer

21. A, p. 28
22. D, p. 28
23. B, p. 28
24. D, p. 29
25. C, p. 29
26. A, p. 28
27. B, p. 30
28. C, p. 30
29. D, p. 30
30. A, p. 32
31. B, p. 30
32. A, p. 30

Circle the one that does *not* belong

33. Uracil (RNA contains the base uracil, not DNA)
34. RNA (the others are complementary base pairings of DNA)
35. Anaphase (the others refer to genes and heredity)
36. Thymine (the others refer to RNA)
37. Interphase (the others refer to translation)
38. Prophase (the others refer to anaphase)
39. Prophase (the others refer to interphase)
40. Metaphase (the others refer to telophase)
41. Gene (the others refer to stages of cell division)

42. Fill in the missing area

TISSUE	LOCATION	FUNCTION
EPITHELIAL		
1.	1A.	1A. Absorption by diffusion of respiratory gases between alveolar air and blood
	1B.	1B. Absorption by diffusion, filtration and osmosis
2.	2A. Surface of lining of mouth and esophagus	2.
	2B. Surface of skin	
3.	3. Surface layer of lining of stomach, intestines, and parts of respiratory tract	3.
4. Stratified transitional	4.	4.
5.	5. Surface of lining of trachea	5.
6.	6.	6. Secretion; absorption
CONNECTIVE		
1.	1. Between other tissues and organs	1.
2. Adipose	2.	2.
3.	3.	3. Flexible but strong connection
4.	4. Skeleton	4.
5.	5. Part of nasal septum, larynx, rings in trachea and bronchi, disks between vertebrae, external ear	5.
6.	6.	6. Transportation
7. Hemopoietic tissue	7.	7.

continued

TISSUE	LOCATION	FUNCTION
MUSCLE		
1.	1. Muscles that attach to bones, eyeball muscles, upper third of esophagus	1.
2. Cardiac	2.	2.
3.	3. Walls of digestive, respiratory, and genitourinary tracts; walls of blood and large lymphatic vessels; ducts of glands; intrinsic eye muscles; arrector muscles of hair	3.
NERVOUS		
1.	1. Brain and spinal cord, nerves	1.

Applying what you know

43.

47. WORD FIND

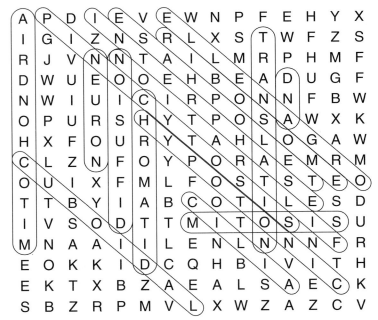

44. Diffusion
45. Absorption of oxygen into Ms. Bence's blood.
46. Merrily may have exceeded the 18% to 24% desirable body fat composition. Fitness depends more on the percentage and ratio of specific tissue types than the overall amount of tissue present.

Crossword puzzle

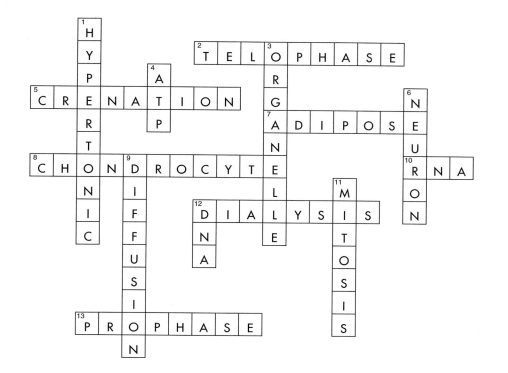

Check your knowledge

MULTIPLE CHOICE

1. A, p. 26
2. B, p. 30
3. B, p. 27
4. C, p. 36
5. C, p. 30
6. A, p. 35
7. A, p. 44
8. B, p. 42
9. C, p. 42
10. D, p. 44

MATCHING

11. F, p. 43
12. G, p. 22
13. J, p. 46
14. C, p. 32
15. A, p. 36
16. B, p. 33
17. I, p. 28
18. H, p. 38
19. D, p. 26
20. E, p. 45

CELL STRUCTURE

MITOSIS

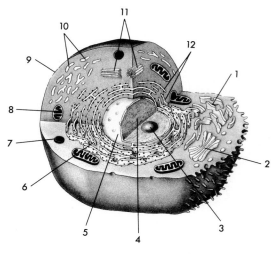

1. Smooth endoplasmic reticulum
2. Golgi apparatus
3. Nucleolus
4. Nucleus
5. Nuclear membrane
6. Rough endoplasmic reticulum
7. Lysosome
8. Mitochondrion
9. Plasma membrane
10. Smooth endoplasmic reticulum
11. Centrioles
12. Ribosomes

1. Interphase
2. Prophase
3. Metaphase
4. Anaphase
5. Telophase
6. Daughter cells (interphase)

278   Answer Key

TISSUES

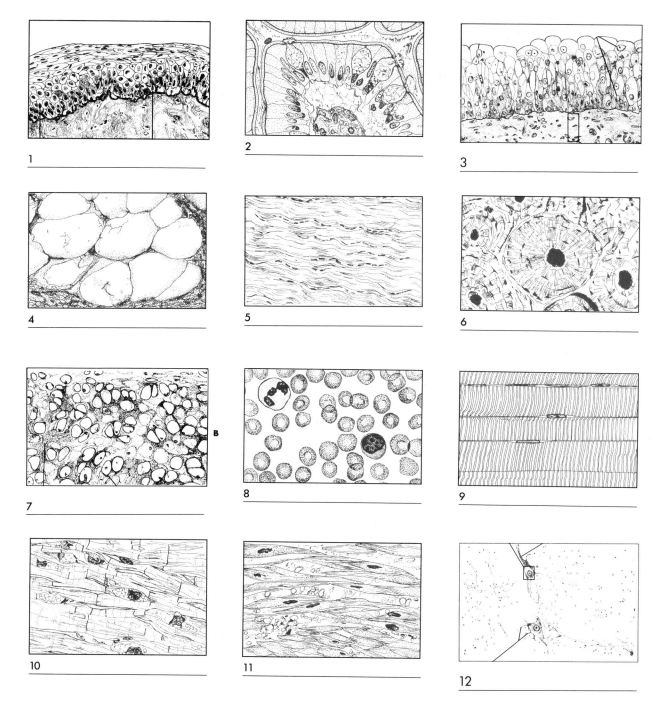

1. _____

2. _____

3. _____

4. _____

5. _____

6. _____

7. _____

8. _____

9. _____

10. _____

11. _____

12. _____

1. Stratified squamous epithelium
2. Simple columnar epithelium
3. Stratified transitional epithelium
4. Adipose tissue
5. Dense fibrous connective tissue
6. Bone tissue
7. Cartilage
8. Blood
9. Skeletal muscle
10. Cardiac muscle
11. Smooth muscle
12. Nervous tissue

CHAPTER 3
ORGAN SYSTEMS OF THE BODY

Matching

1. A, p. 58
2. E, p. 58
3. D, p. 61
4. B, p. 61
5. C, p. 63
6. F, p. 63
7. E, p. 63
8. B, p. 67
9. A, p. 65
10. C, p. 65
11. D, p. 68

Circle the one that does *not* belong

12. Mouth (the others refer to the respiratory system)
13. Rectum (the others refer to the reproductive system)
14. Pancreas (the others refer to the circulatory system)
15. Pineal (the others refer to the urinary system)
16. Joints (the others refer to the muscular system)
17. Pituitary (the others refer to the nervous system)
18. Tendons (the others refer to the skeletal system)
19. Appendix (the others refer to the endocrine system)
20. Thymus (the others refer to the integumentary system)
21. Trachea (the others refer to the digestive system)
22. Liver (the others refer to the lymphatic system)

Fill in the missing area

SYSTEM	ORGAN	FUNCTIONS
23.	23.	23. Protection, regulation of body temperature, synthesis of chemicals and hormones, serves as a sense organ
24.	24. Bones, joints	24.
25.	25.	25. Movement, maintains body posture, produces heat
26. Nervous	26.	26.
27.	27. Pituitary, thymus, pineal, adrenal, hypothalamus, thyroid, pancreas, parathyroid, ovaries, testes	27.
28.	28.	28. Transportation, immunity
29.	29. Lymph nodes, lymph vessels, thymus, spleen, tonsils	29.
30. Urinary	30.	30.
31.	31. Mouth, pharynx, esophagus, stomach, small and large intestine, rectum, anal canal, teeth, salivary glands, tongue, liver, gallbladder, pancreas, appendix	31.
32. Respiratory	32.	32.
33.	33. Gonads—testes and ovaries; accessory glands (p. 72); and supporting structures (p. 72)	33.

Unscramble the words

34. Heart
35. Pineal
36. Nerve
37. Esophagus
38. Nervous

Applying what you know

39. Endocrinology and gynecology
40. The skin protects the underlying tissue against invasion by harmful bacteria. With such a large percentage of his skin destroyed, Brian was vulnerable to bacteria, and so he was placed in the cleanest environment possible-isolation. Jenny is required to wear special attire so that the risk of a visitor bringing bacteria to the patient is reduced.
41. WORD FIND

```
Y  R  A  T  N  E  M  U  G  E  T  N  I  R  F
H  N  E  R  V  O  U  S  K  I  R  J  M  G  T
L  Y  M  P  H  A  T  I  C  I  S  Y  Y  U  I
B  N  X  Y  R  O  T  A  L  U  C  R  I  C  W
P  E  L  R  E  O  M  J  M  S  O  M  M  P  S
C  C  W  M  A  N  D  L  A  T  E  L  E  K  S
R  R  K  E  M  L  I  U  A  V  V  U  K  N
D  K  X  P  D  J  U  R  C  J  I  R  Q  E  M
C  D  B  V  C  V  I  C  C  T  T  K  W  C  X
X  R  Q  Q  D  P  H  C  S  O  I  X  P  A  Z
M  F  M  U  S  Y  D  E  V  U  D  V  Y  K  E
U  E  S  E  C  Z  G  T  Q  D  M  N  E  K  O
P  Y  R  A  N  I  R  U  C  T  C  N  E  W  H
N  H  T  N  D  E  P  S  I  X  A  Q  O  I  E
```

Check your knowledge

MULTIPLE CHOICE

1. D, p. 67
2. C, p. 68
3. C, p. 67
4. B, p. 63
5. D, p. 58
6. A, p. 67
7. B, p. 61
8. A, p. 58
9. A, p. 65
10. C, p. 57

MATCHING

11. C, p. 58
12. D, p. 63
13. H, p. 63
14. G, p. 68
15. B, p. 67
16. F, p. 67
17. I, p. 68
18. E, p. 65
19. J, p. 61
20. A, p. 63

Crossword puzzle

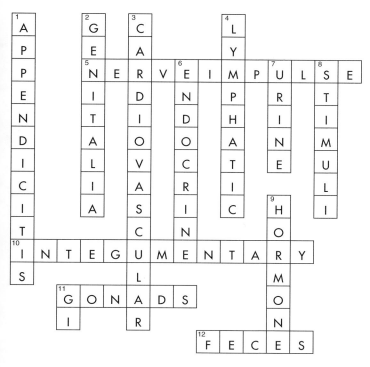

CHAPTER 4
THE INTEGUMENTARY SYSTEM AND BODY MEMBRANES

Select the correct term

1. B, p. 78
2. D, p. 80
3. C, p. 79
4. A, p. 78
5. B, p. 78
6. D, p. 80
7. C, p. 79
8. C, p. 79

Matching

9. D, p. 80
10. A, p. 80
11. B, p. 80
12. C, p. 83
13. E, p. 80
14. A, p. 80
15. D, p. 82
16. E, p. 80
17. C, p. 83
18. B, p. 82

Select the correct term

19. A, p. 80
20. B, p. 83
21. B, p. 83
22. A, p. 82
23. A, p. 80
24. B, p. 82
25. B, p. 83
26. B, p. 83
27. B, p. 83
28. A, p. 82 (Fig. 4-3)

Fill in the blanks

29. Protection, temperature regulation, and sense organ activity, p. 87
30. Melanin, p. 87
31. Lanugo, p. 83
32. Hair papillae, p. 83
33. Lunula, p. 83
34. Arrector pili, p. 84
35. Light touch, p. 88
36. Eccrine, p. 87
37. Apocrine, p. 87
38. Sebum, p. 87

Circle the correct answer

39. Will not, p. 90
40. Will, p. 90
41. Will not, p. 90
42. 11, p. 90
43. Third, p. 90

Unscramble the words

44. Epidermis
45. Keratin
46. Hair
47. Lanugo
48. Dehydration
49. Third degree

Applying what you know

50. 46%
51. Pleurisy
52. Fingerprints
53. WORD FIND

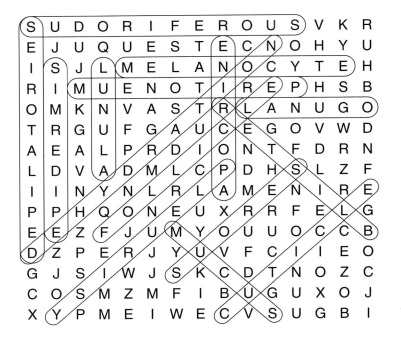

Check your knowledge

MULTIPLE CHOICE

1. A, p. 78
2. B, p. 80
3. A, p. 84
4. D, p. 87
5. B, p. 82
6. D, p. 90
7. B, p. 87
8. B, p. 80
9. C, p. 87
10. B, p. 87

MATCHING

11. C, p. 82
12. D, p. 78
13. B, p. 88
14. G, p. 80
15. I, p. 80
16. H, p. 83
17. J, p. 87
18. E, p. 80
19. A, p. 83
20. F, p. 87

COMPLETION

21. H, p. 87
22. A, p. 80
23. B, p. 87
24. F, p. 90
25. I, p. 83
26. E, p. 80
27. G, p. 78
28. D, p. 79
29. J, p. 88
30. C, p. 78

Crossword puzzle

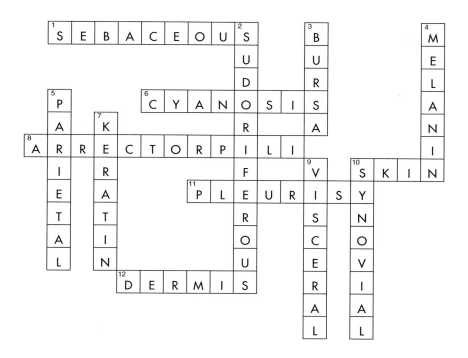

LONGITUDINAL SECTION OF THE SKIN

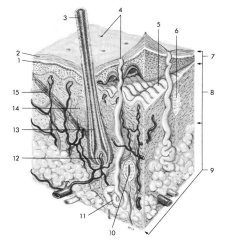

1. Pigment layer
2. Stratum corneum
3. Hair shaft
4. Openings of sweat ducts
5. Dermal papilla
6. Meissner's corpuscle
7. Epidermis
8. Dermis

9. Subcutaneous fatty tissue
10. Pacinian corpuscle
11. Sweat gland
12. Papilla of hair
13. Hair follicle
14. Sebaceous (oil) gland
15. Arrector pili muscle

"RULE OF NINES" FOR ESTIMATING SKIN SURFACE BURNED

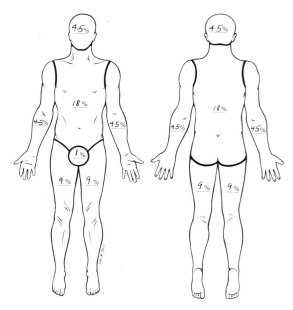

CHAPTER 5
THE SKELETAL SYSTEM

Fill in the blanks

1. 4, p. 98
2. Medullary cavity, p. 98
3. Articular cartilage p. 98
4. Endosteum, p. 99
5. Hemopoiesis, p. 98
6. Red bone marrow, p. 98
7. Periosteum, p. 99
8. Elderly white female, p. 103
9. Calcium, p. 98
10. Move, p. 98

Matching

11. D, p. 99
12. B, p. 99
13. E, p. 99
14. A, p. 99
15. C, p. 99
16. D, p. 99
17. A, p. 99
18. E, p. 99
19. B. p. 101
20. C, p. 99

True or false

21. T
22. Epiphyses, not diaphyses, p. 101
23. Osteoblasts, not osteoclasts, p. 101
24. T
25. Increase, not decrease, p. 101
26. Juvenile, not adult, p. 103
27. Diaphysis, not articulation, p. 101
28. T
29. Ceases, not begins, p. 103
30. T

Circle the correct answer

31. A, p. 104
32. D, p. 107
33. A, p. 111
34. D, p. 111
35. C, p. 114
36. C, p. 115
37. D, p. 114
38. D, p. 114
39. A, p. 115
40. B, p. 107
41. A, p. 111
42. B, p. 114
43. B, p. 111
44. B, p. 114
45. C, p. 114
46. A, p. 115
47. D, p. 107
48. C, p. 110
49. C, p. 107

Circle the one that does *not* belong

50. Coxal bone (all others refer to the spine)
51. Axial (all others refer to the appendicular skeleton)
52. Maxilla, (all others refer to the cranial bones)
53. Ribs (all others refer to the shoulder girdle)
54. Vomer (all others refer to the bones of the middle ear)
55. Ulna (all others refer to the coxal bone)
56. Ethmoid (all others refer to the hand and wrist)
57. Nasal (all others refer to cranial bones)
58. Anvil (all others refer to the cervical vertebra)

Select the correct term

59. A, p. 119
60. B, p. 119
61. B, p. 103
62. A, p. 118
63. B, p. 119

Matching

64. C, p. 107
65. G, p. 112
66. J, L, M and K, p. 117
67. N, p. 117
68. I, p. 114
69. A, p. 107
70. P, p. 117
71. D, B, p. 107
72. F, p. 107
73. H, Q, p. 114
74. O, T, p. 117
75. R, p. 107
76. S, E, p. 107

Circle the correct answer

77. Diarthroses, p. 120
78. Synarthrotic, p. 120
79. Diarthrotic, p. 121
80. Ligaments, p. 121
81. Articular cartilage, p. 121
82. Least movable, p. 121
83. Largest, p. 126
84. 2, p. 122
85. Mobility, p. 122
86. Pivot, p. 122

Unscramble the words

87. Vertebrae
88. Pubis
89. Scapula
90. Mandible
91. Phalanges
92. Pelvic girdle

Applying what you know

93. The bones are responsible for the majority of our blood cell formation. The disease condition of the bones might be inhibiting the production of blood cells for Mrs. Perine.
94. Epiphyseal cartilage is present only while a child is still growing. It becomes bone in adulthood. It is particularly vulnerable to fractures in childhood and preadolescence.
95. Osteoporosis

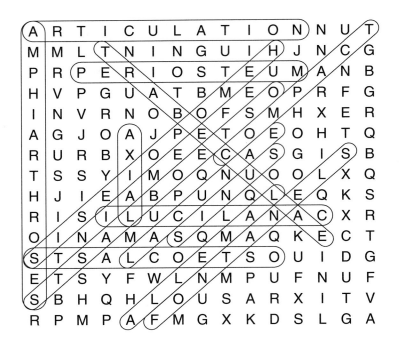

Crossword puzzle

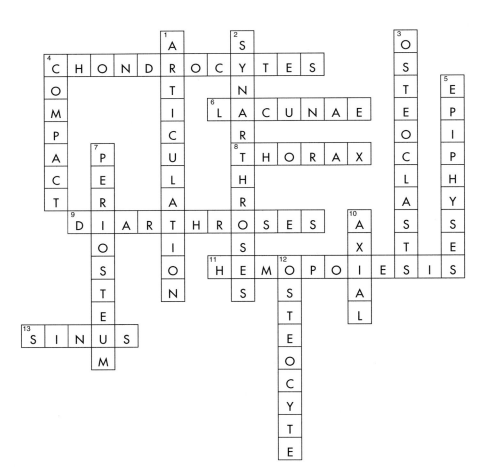

Check your knowledge

MULTIPLE CHOICE

1. A, p. 111
2. C, p. 114
3. A, p. 98
4. C, p. 118
5. C, p. 111
6. D, p. 121
7. C, p. 104
8. C, p. 107
9. D, p. 101
10. A, p. 120

MATCHING

11. G, p. 121
12. B, p. 99
13. I, p. 120
14. J, p. 107
15. E, p. 117
16. H, p. 101
17. A, p. 99
18. C, p. 107
19. F, p. 117
20. D, p. 98

LONGITUDINAL SECTION OF LONG BONE

1. Articular cartilage
2. Spongy bone
3. Epiphyseal plate
4. Red marrow cavities
5. Compact bone
6. Medullary cavity
7. Yellow marrow
8. Periosteum

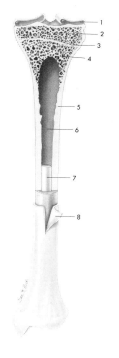

ANTERIOR VIEW OF SKELETON

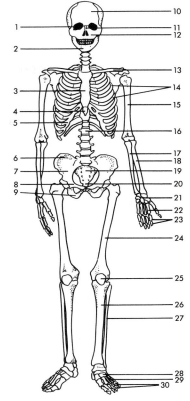

1. Orbit
2. Mandible
3. Sternum
4. Xiphoid process
5. Costal cartilage
6. Coxal
7. Ilium
8. Pubis
9. Ischium
10. Frontal
11. Nasal
12. Maxilla
13. Clavicle
14. Ribs
15. Humerus
16. Vertebral column
17. Ulna
18. Radius
19. Sacrum
20. Coccyx
21. Carpals
22. Metacarpals
23. Phalanges
24. Femur
25. Patella

26. Tibia
27. Fibula
28. Tarsals
29. Metatarsals
30. Phalanges

POSTERIOR VIEW OF SKELETON

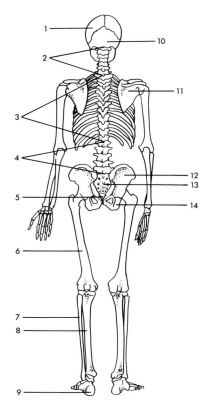

1. Parietal
2. Cervical vertebrae
3. Thoracic vertebrae
4. Lumbar vertebrae
5. Coccyx
6. Femur
7. Fibula
8. Tibia
9. Calcaneus
10. Occipital
11. Scapula
12. Coxal (hip) bone
13. Sacrum
14. Ischium

SKULL VIEWED FROM THE RIGHT SIDE

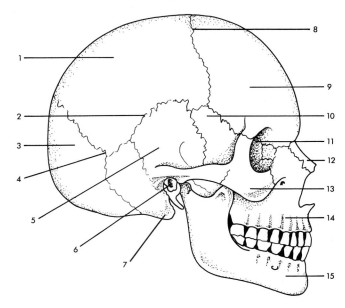

1. Parietal bone
2. Squamous suture
3. Occipital bone
4. Lambdoidal suture
5. Temporal bone
6. External auditory canal
7. Mastoid process
8. Coronal suture
9. Frontal bone
10. Sphenoid bone
11. Ethmoid bone
12. Nasal bone
13. Zygomatic bone
14. Maxilla
15. Mandible

SKULL VIEWED FROM THE FRONT

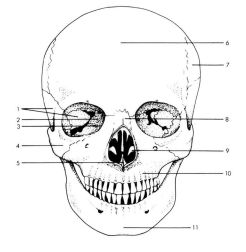

1. Sphenoid bone
2. Ethmoid bone
3. Lacrimal bone
4. Zygomatic bone
5. Vomer
6. Frontal bone
7. Parietal bone
8. Nasal bone
9. Inferior concha
10. Maxilla
11. Mandible

STRUCTURE OF A DIARTHROTIC JOINT

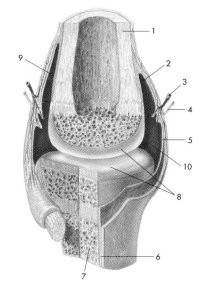

1. Bone
2. Synovial membrane
3. Blood vessel
4. Nerve
5. Joint capsule
6. Periosteum
7. Bone
8. Articular cartilage
9. Bursa
10. Joint cavity

CHAPTER 6
THE MUSCULAR SYSTEM

Select the correct term
1. A, p. 134
2. B, p. 134
3. C, p. 135
4. C, p. 134
5. A, p. 134
6. B, p. 135
7. C and B, p. 134
8. A, p. 134
9. C, p. 134
10. C, p. 135

Matching
11. D, p. 135
12. B, p. 135
13. A, p. 135
14. E, p. 135
15. C, p. 135
16. E, p. 135
17. C, p. 135
18. B, p. 135
19. A, p. 135
20. D, p. 135

Fill in the blanks
21. Pulling, p. 137
22. Insertion, p. 137
23. Insertion, origin, p. 137
24. Prime mover, p. 137
25. Antagonists, p. 137
26. Synergist, p. 137
27. Tonic contraction, p. 138
28. Muscle tone, p. 138
29. Hypothermia, p. 138
30. ATP, p. 138

True or false
31. Neuromuscular junction, p. 139
32. T
33. T
34. Oxygen debt, p. 138
35. "All or none", p. 140
36. Lactic acid, p. 138
37. T
38. T
39. Skeletal muscle, p. 138
40. T

Circle the correct answer
41. A, p. 140
42. B, p. 140
43. B, p. 140
44. C, p. 141
45. D, p. 140
46. A, p. 140
47. B, p. 140
48. C, p. 140
49. B, p. 140
50. D, p. 140

Choose the proper function or functions for the muscles listed below

51. C, p. 145
52. F, p. 150, and A and D, p. 153
53. F, p. 153, and B, p. 146
54. A, p. 145
55. C, p. 153
56. B, p. 153, and F, p. 146
57. A, p. 145
58. A and D, p. 145
59. B, p. 145
60. B, p. 145
61. A, p. 147, and E, p. 145
62. B, p. 145
63. D, p. 145

Circle the correct answer

64. A, p. 150
65. D, p. 150
66. C, p. 150
67. A, p. 150
68. D, p. 150
69. C, p. 150

Applying what you know

70. Bursitis
71. Deltoid area
72. Tendon
73. WORD FIND

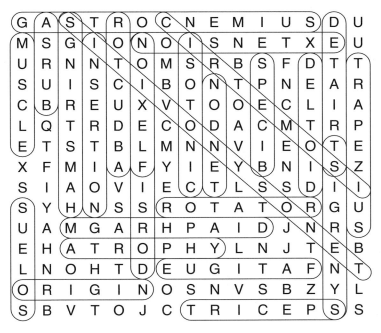

Crossword puzzle

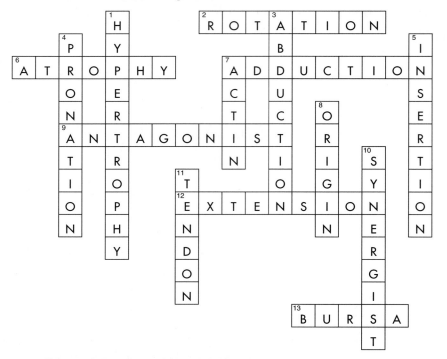

Check your knowledge

MULTIPLE CHOICE

1. D, p. 139
2. A, p. 150
3. C, p. 137
4. B, p. 146
5. A, p. 140
6. B, p. 138
7. D, p. 140
8. A, p. 140
9. A, p. 140
10. C, p. 135

TRUE OR FALSE

11. T
12. T
13. F (pronation)
14. F (hypertrophy)
15. T
16. T
17. T
18. F (hypothermia)
19. T
20. F (flexion)

MUSCLES ANTERIOR VIEW

1. Sternocleidomastoid
2. Trapezius
3. Pectoralis major
4. Rectus abdominis
5. External abdominal oblique
6. Iliopsoas
7. Quadriceps group
8. Tibialis anterior
9. Peroneus longus
10. Peroneus brevis
11. Soleus
12. Gastrocnemius
13. Sartorius
14. Adductor group
15. Brachialis
16. Biceps brachii
17. Deltoid
18. Facial muscles

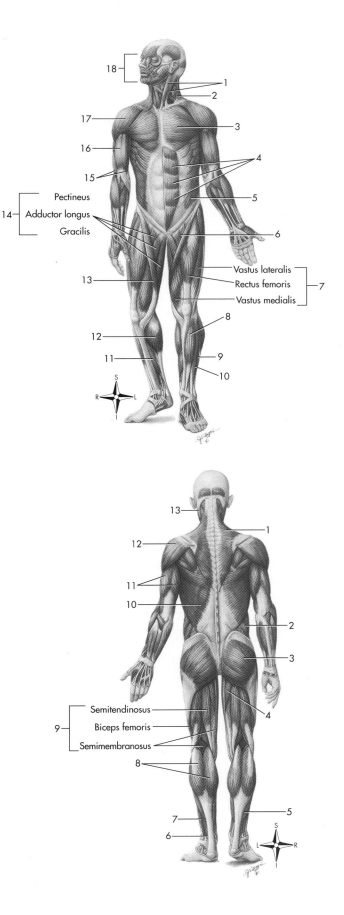

MUSCLES POSTERIOR VIEW

1. Trapezius
2. External abdominal oblique
3. Gluteus maximus
4. Adductor magnus
5. Soleus
6. Peroneus brevis
7. Peroneus longus
8. Gastrocnemius
9. Hamstring group
10. Latissimus dorsi
11. Triceps brachii
12. Deltoid
13. Sternocleidomastoid

CHAPTER 7
THE NERVOUS SYSTEM

Matching

1. B. p. 164
2. C, p. 165
3. D, p. 165
4. A, p. 165
5. B, p. 165
6. D, p. 165
7. C, p. 165
8. A, p. 165
9. F, p. 167
10. E, p. 167

Select the correct term

11. A, p. 165
12. B, p. 165
13. B, p. 165
14. A, p. 165
15. A, p. 165
16. B, p. 165
17. B, p. 167
18. A, p. 165
19. B, p. 170
20. A, p. 165

Fill in the blanks

21. Two-neuron arc, p. 168
22. Sensory, interneurons, motor neurons, p. 168
23. Receptors, p. 169
24. Synapse, p. 169
25. Reflex, p. 169

26. Withdrawal reflex, p. 170
27. Ganglion, p. 169
28. Interneurons, p. 170
29. Knee jerk, p. 169
30. Gray matter, p. 170

Circle the correct answer

31. Do not, p. 171
32. Increases, p. 171
33. Excess, p. 171
34. Postsynaptic, p. 171
35. Presynaptic, p. 171
36. Neurotransmitter, p. 171
37. Communicate, p. 171
38. Specifically, p. 171
39. Sleep, p. 171
40. Pain, p. 173

Circle the correct answer

41. E, p. 174
42. D, p. 174
43. A, p. 176
44. E, p. 176
45. E, p. 176
46. D, p. 176
47. B, p. 177
48. E, p. 177
49. B, p. 177
50. D, p. 177
51. D, p. 177
52. B, p. 177
53. A, p. 177
54. D, p. 179
55. C, p. 177

True or false

56. 17 to 18 inches, p. 179
57. Bottom of the first lumbar vertebra, p. 179
58. Lumbar punctures, p. 183
59. Spinal tracts, p. 179
60. T
61. One general function, p. 179
62. Anesthesia, p. 180

Circle the one that does *not* belong

63. Ventricles (all others refer to meninges)
64. CSF (all others refer to the arachnoid)
65. Pia mater (all others refer to the cerebrospinal fluid)
66. Choroid plexus (all others refer to the dura mater)
67. Brain tumor (all others refer to a lumbar puncture)

68. Fill in the missing areas on the chart below.

CRANIAL NERVES

Nerve	Conduct Impulses	Function
I Olfactory		
II		Vision
III	From brain to eye muscles	
IV Trochlear		
V		Sensations of face, scalp, and teeth, chewing movements
VI	From brain to external eye muscles	
VII		Sense of taste; contractions of muscles of facial expression
VIII Vestibulocochlear		
IX	From throat and taste buds of tongue to brain; also from brain to throat muscles and salivary glands	
X Vagus		
XI		Shoulder movements; turning movements of head
XII Hypoglossal		

Select the correct term

69. A, p. 186
70. B, p. 186
71. A, p. 186
72. B, p. 195
73. B, p. 186
74. A, p. 186
75. B, p. 186
76. B, p. 186

Matching

77. D, p. 188
78. E, p. 189
79. F, p. 189
80. B, p. 189
81. A, p. 188
82. C, p. 188

Circle the correct answer

83. C, p. 191
84. B, p. 191
85. B, p. 193
86. D, p. 192
87. A, p. 193
88. A, p. 193

Select the correct term

89. B, p. 192
90. A, p. 192
91. A, p. 192
92. B, p. 192
93. A, p. 192
94. B, p. 192
95. A, p. 192
96. A, p. 192
97. B, p. 192
98. B, p. 192

Fill in the blanks

99. Acetylcholine, p. 194
100. Adrenergic fibers, p. 194
101. Cholinergic fibers, p. 194
102. Homeostasis, p. 194
103. Heart rate, p. 194
104. Decreased, p. 194

Unscramble the words

105. Neurons
106. Synapse
107. Autonomic
108. Smooth muscle
109. Sympathetic

Applying what you know

110. Right
111. Hydrocephalus
112. Sympathetic
113. Parasympathetic
114. Sympathetic; No, he shouldn't, because the digestive process is not active during sympathetic control. Bill may experience nausea, vomiting or discomfort because of this factor. See p. 192

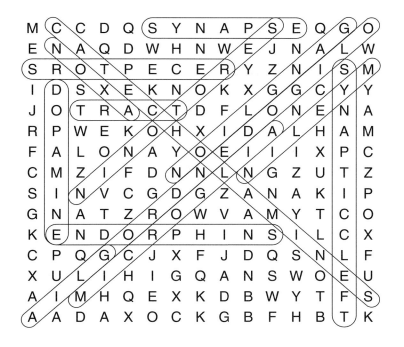

Crossword puzzle

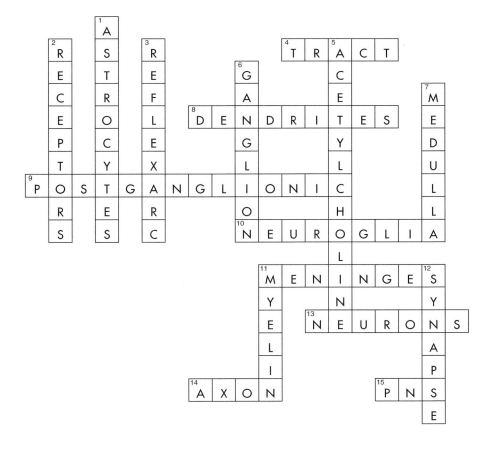

Check your knowledge

MULTIPLE CHOICE

1. D, p. 165
2. B, p. 182
3. A, p. 182
4. B, p. 177
5. A, p. 192
6. D, p. 194
7. D, p. 165
8. C, p. 171
9. C, p. 179
10. D, p. 194

MATCHING

11. C, p. 167
12. A, p. 165
13. J, p. 174
14. H, p. 171
15. B, p. 168
16. I, p. 186
17. F, p. 165
18. E, p. 176
19. D, p. 186
20. G, p. 179

NEURON

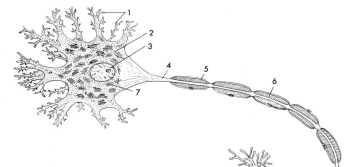

1. Dendrites
2. Cell body
3. Nucleus
4. Axon
5. Schwann cell
6. Myelin
7. Mitochondrion

CRANIAL NERVES

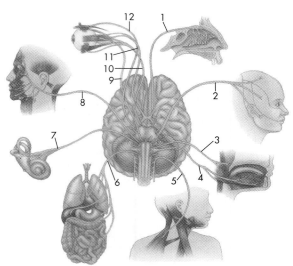

1. Olfactory nerve
2. Trigeminal nerve
3. Glossopharyngeal nerve
4. Hypoglossal nerve
5. Accessory nerve
6. Vagus nerve
7. Vestibulocochlear nerve
8. Facial nerve
9. Abducens nerve
10. Oculomotor nerve
11. Optic nerve
12. Trochlear nerve

NEURAL PATHWAY INVOLVED IN THE PATELLAR REFLEX

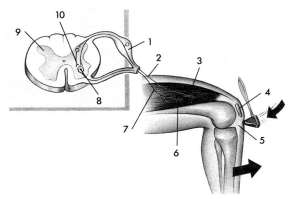

1. Dorsal root ganglion
2. Sensory neuron
3. Stretch receptor
4. Patella
5. Patellar tendon
6. Quadriceps muscle
7. Motor neuron
8. Monosynaptic synapse
9. Gray matter
10. Interneuron

THE CEREBRUM

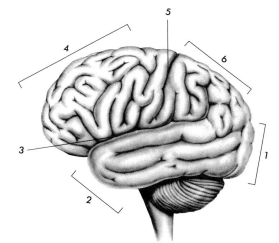

1. Occipital lobe
2. Temporal lobe
3. Lateral fissure
4. Frontal lobe
5. Central sulcus
6. Parietal lobe

SAGITTAL SECTION OF THE CENTRAL NERVOUS SYSTEM

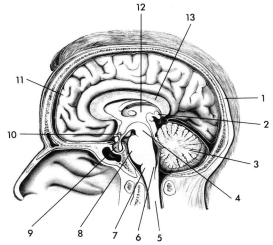

1. Skull
2. Pineal gland
3. Cerebellum
4. Midbrain
5. Spinal cord
6. Medulla
7. Reticular formation
8. Pons
9. Pituitary gland
10. Hypothalamus
11. Cerebral cortex
12. Thalamus
13. Corpus callosum

NEURON PATHWAYS

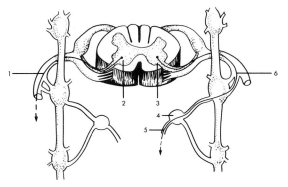

1. Somatic motor neuron's axon
2. Cell body of somatic motor neuron
3. Cell body of preganglionic neuron
4. Collateral ganglion
5. Postganglionic neuron's axon
6. Preganglionic sympathetic neuron's axon

Answer Key   301

CHAPTER 8
SENSE ORGANS

Matching

1. D, p. 204
2. B, p. 204
3. A, p. 206
4. E, p. 206
5. C, p. 206

Circle the correct answer

6. C, p. 204
7. E, p. 207
8. B, p. 207
9. C, p. 207
10. E, p. 207
11. D, p. 207
12. A, p. 207
13. B, p. 207
14. C, p. 209
15. B, p. 210
16. D, p. 208
17. A, p. 208
18. D, p. 211

Select the correct term

19. B, p. 214
20. C, p. 214
21. B, p. 214
22. A, p. 214
23. C, p. 214
24. A, p. 213
25. C, p. 214
26. B, p. 214
27. B, p. 214
28. C, p. 214

Fill in the blanks

29. Auricle, external auditory canal, p. 213
30. Eardrum, p. 213
31. Ossicles, p. 214
32. Oval window, p. 214
33. Otitis media, p. 214
34. Vestibule, p. 214
35. Mechanoreceptors, p. 214
36. Crista ampullaris, p. 214

Circle the correct answer

37. Papillae, p. 215
38. Cranial, p. 217
39. Mucus, p. 217
40. Memory, p. 218
41. Chemoreceptors, p. 214

Unscramble the words

42. Auricle
43. Sclera
44. Papilla
45. Conjunctiva
46. Pupils

Applying what you know

47. External otitis
48. Cataracts
49. The eustachian tube connects the throat to the middle ear and provides a perfect pathway for the spread of infection.
50. Olfactory

51. WORD FIND

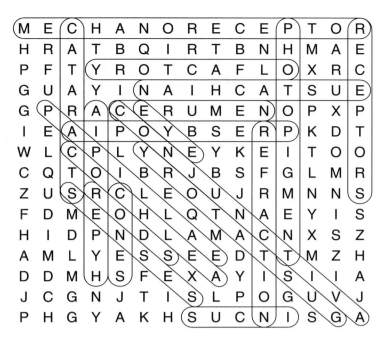

Crossword puzzle

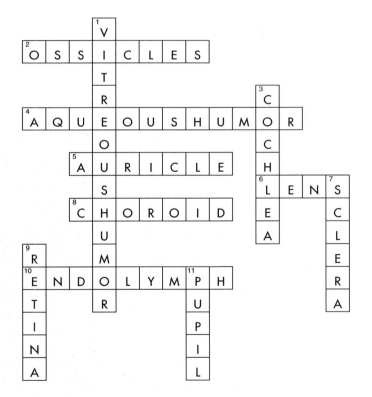

Check your knowledge

EYE

MULTIPLE CHOICE

1. A, p. 214
2. B, p. 214
3. A, p. 217
4. C, p. 209
5. B, p. 204
6. B, p. 205
7. D, p. 204
8. B, p. 207
9. D, p. 217
10. A, p. 213

TRUE OR FALSE

11. T
12. Aqueous humor
13. T
14. Semicircular canals
15. T
16. T
17. T
18. T
19. T
20. T

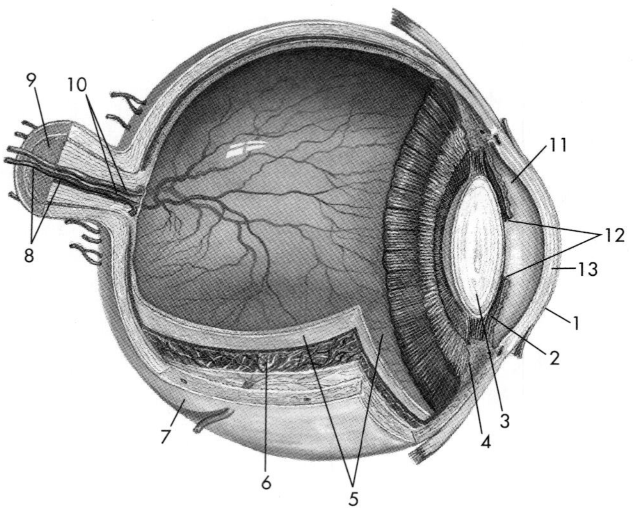

1. Conjunctiva
2. Iris
3. Lens
4. Ciliary muscle
5. Retina
6. Choroid layer
7. Sclera
8. Central retinal artery and vein
9. Optic nerve
10. Optic disc (blind spot)
11. Anterior cavity
12. Pupil
13. Cornea

EAR

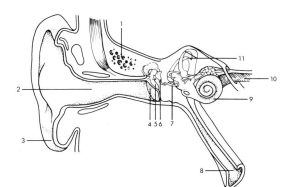

1. Temporal bone
2. External auditory meatus
3. Auricle (pinna)
4. Tympanic membrane (eardrum)
5. Malleus
6. Incus
7. Stapes
8. Auditory (Eustachian tube)
9. Cochlea
10. Cochlear nerve
11. Semicircular canals

CHAPTER 9
ENDOCRINE SYSTEM

Matching

1. D, p. 226
2. C, p. 226
3. E, p. 226
4. A, p. 226
5. B, p. 226
6. E, p. 229
7. C, p. 231
8. A, p. 226
9. D, p. 225
10. B, p. 226

Fill in the blanks

11. Second messenger, p. 226
12. Recognize, p. 226
13. First messengers, p. 229
14. Target organs, p. 229
15. Cyclic AMP, p. 229
16. Target cells, p. 229
17. G protein, nitric oxide, p. 229

Circle the correct answer

18. B, p. 232
19. E, p. 232
20. D, p. 232
21. D, p. 233
22. A, p. 233
23. C, p. 233
24. C, p. 233
25. B, p. 232
26. A, p. 232
27. A, p. 232
28. D, p. 233
29. B, p. 233
30. A, p. 233
31. C, p. 233
32. C, p. 234

Select the correct term

33. A, p. 231
34. B, p. 231
35. B, p. 233
36. C, p. 235
37. A, p. 232
38. C, p. 235
39. A, p. 233
40. A, p. 232
41. A, p. 232
42. C, p. 234

Circle the correct answer

43. Below, p. 235
44. Calcitonin, p. 235
45. Iodine, p. 235
46. Do not, p. 235
47. Thyroid, p. 235
48. Decreases, p. 236
49. Hypothyroidism, p. 237
50. Cretinism, p. 237
51. PTH, p. 236
52. Increase, p. 236

Fill in the blanks

53. Adrenal cortex, adrenal medulla, p. 236
54. Corticoids, p. 237
55. Mineralocorticoids, p. 237
56. Glucocorticoids, p. 237
57. Sex hormones, p. 237
58. Gluconeogenesis, p. 238
59. Blood pressure, p. 238
60. Epinephrine, norepinephrine, p. 240
61. Stress, p. 240
62. Addison's disease, p. 241

Select the correct term

63. A, p. 237
64. A, p. 239
65. B, p. 241
66. A, p. 241
67. B, p. 240
68. A, p. 237
69. A, p. 240

Circle the term that does *not* belong

70. Beta cells (all others refer to glucagon)
71. Glucagon (all others refer to insulin)
72. Thymosin (all others refer to female sex glands)
73. Chorion (all other refer to male sex glands)
74. Aldosterone (all others refer to the thymus)
75. ACTH (all others refer to the placenta)
76. Semen (all others refer to the pineal gland)

Matching

77. E, p. 242
78. C, p. 242
79. B, p. 245
80. D, p. 245
81. A, p. 245
82. E, p. 245
83. A, p. 245
84. B, p. 246
85. C, p. 245
86. D, p. 245

Unscramble the words

87. Corticoids
88. Diuresis
89. Glucocorticoids
90. Steroids
91. Stress

Applying what you know

92. She was pregnant
93. Zona reticularis of the adrenal cortex
94. Oxytocin
95. WORD FIND

Crossword puzzle

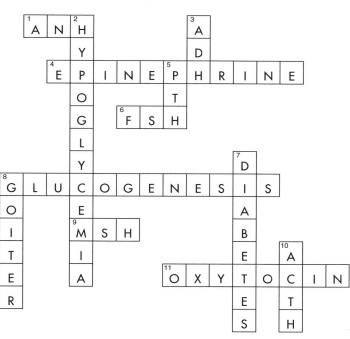

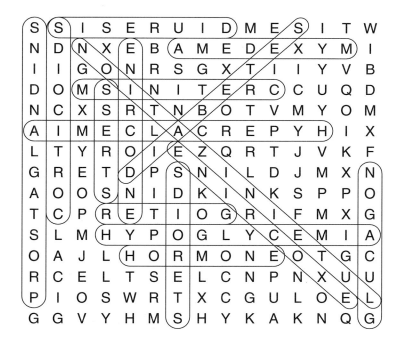

Check your knowledge

MULTIPLE CHOICE

1. A, p. 237
2. C, p. 233
3. D, p. 237
4. B, p. 232
5. D, p. 245
6. D, p. 233
7. B, p. 245
8. D, p. 227
9. D, p. 242
10. B, p. 231

MATCHING

11. J, p. 237
12. G, p. 233
13. H, p. 242
14. I, p. 227
15. B, p. 233
16. F, p. 245
17. A, p. 241
18. D, p. 233
19. E, p. 232
20. C, p. 236

ENDOCRINE GLANDS

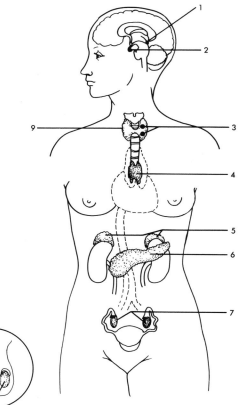

1. Pineal
2. Pituitary
3. Parathyroids
4. Thymus
5. Adrenal
6. Pancreas
7. Ovaries
8. Testes
9. Thyroid

CHAPTER 10
BLOOD

Multiple choice

1. E, p. 256
2. D, p. 257
3. D, p. 257
4. B, p. 257
5. C, p. 257
6. A, p. 258
7. B, p. 259
8. D, p. 257
9. C, p. 261
10. D, p. 258
11. A, p. 259
12. B, p. 265
13. B, p. 262
14. B, p. 257
15. E, p. 257
16. B, p. 257
17. C, p. 257
18. D, p. 257
19. D, p. 259
20. D, p. 259
21. B, p. 261
22. D, p. 258
23. B, p. 260
24. C, p. 260
25. B, p. 260
26. A, p. 262
27. E, p. 262

Fill in the missing areas of the chart

28. p. 264 and 268

Blood Type	Antigen Present in RBCs	Antibody Present in Plasma
A	A	
B		Anti-A
AB	A,B	
O		Anti-A, Anti-B

Fill in the blanks

29. Antigen, p. 262
30. Antibody, p. 264
31. Agglutinate, p. 264
32. Erythroblastosis fetalis, p. 265
33. Rhesus monkeys, p. 265
34. RhoGAM, p. 265
35. AB, p. 265

Applying what you know

36. No. If Mrs. Payne had a negative Rh factor and her husband had a positive Rh factor, it would set up the strong possibility of erythroblastosis fetalis.
37. Both procedures assist the clotting process.

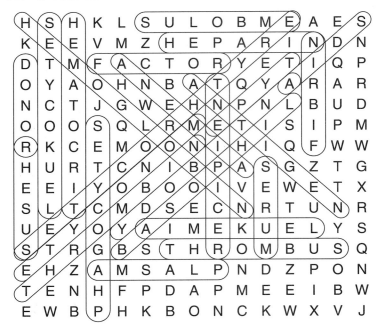

Crossword puzzle

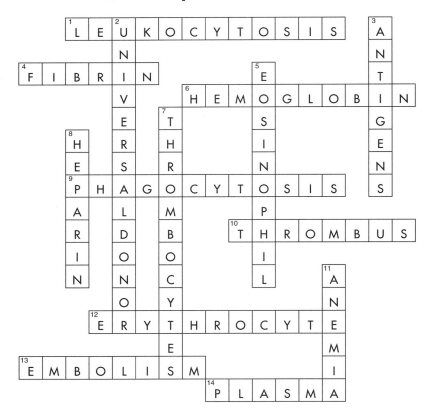

Check your knowledge

MULTIPLE CHOICE

1. B, p. 261
2. B, p. 258
3. A, p. 258
4. A, p. 257
5. D, p. 256
6. A, p. 261
7. A, p. 262
8. D, p. 265
9. C, p. 258
10. B, p. 263

MATCHING

11. D, p. 260
12. F, p. 258
13. H, p. 265
14. A, p. 261
15. G, p. 261
16. C, p. 262
17. B, p. 265
18. E, p. 265
19. I, p. 257
20. J, p. 260

HUMAN BLOOD CELLS

1. Red blood cells
2. Platelets
3. Basophil
4. Neutrophil
5. Eosinophil
6. Lymphocyte
7. Monocyte

BLOOD TYPING

Recipient's blood		Reactions with donor's blood			
RBC antigens	Plasma antibodies	Donor type O	Donor type A	Donor type B	Donor type AB
None (Type O)	Anti-A Anti-B				
A (Type A)	Anti-B				
B (Type B)	Anti-A				
AB (Type AB)	(none)				

Normal blood   Agglutinated blood

CHAPTER 11
THE CIRCULATORY SYSTEM

Fill in the blanks

1. CPR, p. 274
2. Interatrial septum, p. 274
3. Atria, p. 274
4. Ventricles, p. 274
5. Myocardium, p. 274
6. Endocarditis, p. 274
7. Bicuspid or mitral, tricuspid, p. 277
8. Pulmonary circulation, p. 279
9. Coronary embolism or coronary thrombosis, p. 279
10. Myocardial infarction, p. 279
11. Sinoatrial, p. 281
12. P, QRS complex, T, p. 283
13. Repolarization, p. 283

Choose the correct term

14. A, p. 274
15. K, p. 274
16. G, p. 279
17. C, p. 279
18. D, p. 277
19. F, p. 274
20. H, p. 279
21. B, p. 279
22. E, p. 282
23. I, p. 279
24. J, p. 283
25. L, p. 274
26. M, p. 277

Matching

27. D, p. 285
28. B, p. 285
29. C, p. 285
30. G, p. 285
31. A, p. 287
32. E, p. 285
33. F, p. 285

Circle the correct answer

34. D, p. 292
35. C, p. 292
36. B, p. 287
37. A, p. 285
38. B, p. 285
39. B, p. 290
40. D, p. 291
41. B, p. 292
42. B, p. 293
43. A, p. 293
44. D, p. 287
45. A, p. 287

True or false

46. Highest in arteries, lowest in veins, p. 295
47. Blood pressure gradient, p. 295
48. Stop, p. 296
49. High, p. 296
50. Decreases, p. 296
51. T

52. T
53. T
54. Stronger will increase, weaker will decrease, p. 296
55. Contract, p. 298
56. Relax, p. 298
57. Artery, p. 298
58. T
59. T
60. Brachial, p. 298

Unscramble the words
61. Systemic
62. Venule
63. Artery
64. Pulse
65. Vessel

Applying what you know
66. Coronary bypass surgery
67. Artificial pacemaker
68. The endocardial lining can become rough and abrasive to red blood cells passing over its surface. As a result, a fatal blood clot may be formed.
69. Mr. Philbrick may be hemorrhaging. The heart beats faster during hemorrhage in an attempt to compensate for blood loss.

70. WORD FIND

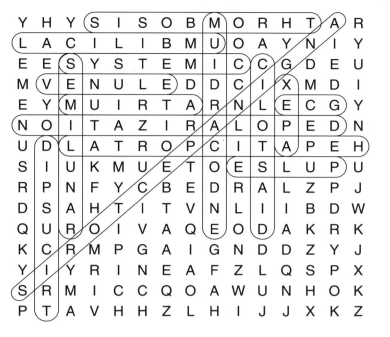

Crossword puzzle

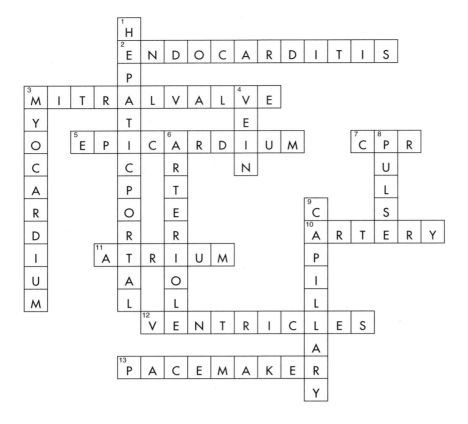

Check your knowledge

MULTIPLE CHOICE

1. A, p. 290
2. C, p. 274
3. B, p. 274
4. A, p. 297
5. A, p. 285
6. D, p. 283
7. C, p. 293
8. D, p. 277
9. C, p. 292
10. C, p. 286

MATCHING

11. F, p. 279
12. G, p. 283
13. H, p. 277
14. I, p. 279
15. J, p. 277
16. B, p. 290
17. C, p. 274
18. A, p. 281
19. D, p. 285
20. E, p. 279

THE HEART

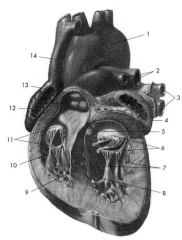

1. Aorta
2. Pulmonary arteries
3. Left pulmonary veins
4. Left atrium
5. Aortic semilunar valve
6. Bicuspid valve
7. Chordae tendineae
8. Left ventricle
9. Interventricular septum
10. Right ventricle
11. Tricuspid valve
12. Right atrium
13. Pulmonary semilunar valve
14. Superior vena cava

CONDUCTION SYSTEM OF THE HEART

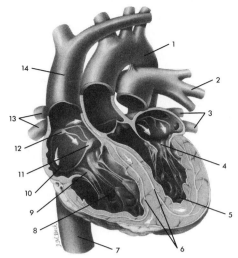

1. Aorta
2. Pulmonary artery
3. Pulmonary veins
4. Mitral (bicuspid) valve
5. Left ventricle
6. Right and left branches of AV bundle
7. Inferior vena cava
8. Right ventricle
9. Tricuspid valve
10. Right atrium
11. Atrioventricular node (AV node)
12. Sinoatrial node (SA node or pacemaker)
13. Pulmonary veins
14. Superior vena cava

FETAL CIRCULATION

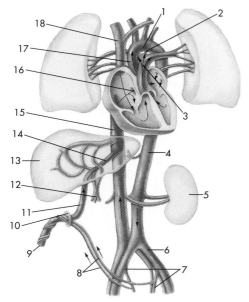

1. Aortic arch
2. Ductus arteriosus
3. Pulmonary trunk
4. Abdominal aorta
5. Kidney
6. Common iliac artery
7. Internal iliac artery
8. Umbilical arteries
9. Umbilical cord
10. Fetal umbilicus
11. Umbilical vein
12. Hepatic portal vein
13. Liver
14. Ductus venosus
15. Inferior vena cava
16. Foramen ovale
17. Ascending aorta
18. Superior vena cava

HEPATIC PORTAL CIRCULATION

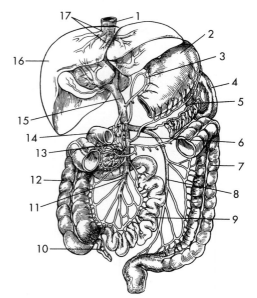

1. Inferior vena cava
2. Stomach
3. Gastric vein
4. Spleen
5. Splenic vein
6. Gastroepiploic vein
7. Descending colon
8. Inferior mesenteric vein
9. Small intestine
10. Appendix
11. Ascending colon
12. Superior mesenteric vein
13. Pancreas
14. Duodenum
15. Hepatic portal vein
16. Liver
17. Hepatic veins

PRINCIPAL ARTERIES OF THE BODY

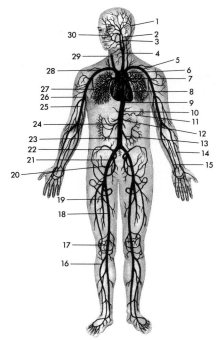

1. Occipital
2. Internal carotid
3. External carotid
4. Left common carotid
5. Left subclavian
6. Arch of aorta
7. Pulmonary
8. Left coronary
9. Aorta
10. Celiac
11. Splenic
12. Renal
13. Inferior mesenteric
14. Radial
15. Ulnar
16. Anterior tibial
17. Popliteal
18. Femoral
19. Deep femoral
20. External iliac
21. Internal iliac
22. Common iliac
23. Abdominal aorta
24. Superior mesenteric
25. Brachial
26. Axillary
27. Right coronary
28. Brachiocephalic
29. Right common carotid
30. Facial

PRINCIPAL VEINS OF THE BODY

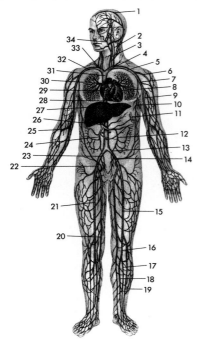

1. Superior sagittal sinus
2. External jugular
3. Internal jugular
4. Left brachiocephalic
5. Left subclavian
6. Cephalic
7. Axillary
8. Great cardiac
9. Basilic
10. Long thoracic
11. Splenic
12. Inferior mesenteric
13. Common iliac
14. Internal iliac
15. Femoral
16. Popliteal
17. Peroneal
18. Anterior tibial
19. Posterior tibial
20. Great saphenous
21. Femoral
22. External iliac
23. Common iliac
24. Superior mesenteric
25. Median cubital
26. Hepatic portal
27. Hepatic
28. Inferior vena cava
29. Small cardiac
30. Pulmonary (right)
31. Superior vena cava
32. Right subclavian
33. Right brachiocephalic
34. Facial

318   Answer Key

NORMAL ECG DEFLECTIONS

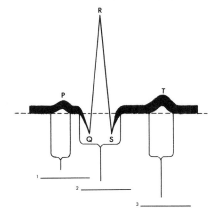

1. Atrial depolarization
2. Ventricular depolarization
3. Ventricular repolarization

CHAPTER 12
THE LYMPHATIC SYSTEM AND IMMUNITY

Fill in the blanks

1. Lymph, p. 308
2. Interstitial fluid, p. 308
3. Lymphatic capillaries, p. 308
4. Right lymphatic duct, thoracic duct, p. 309
5. Cisterna chyli, p. 309
6. Lymph nodes, p. 309
7. Afferent, p. 310
8. Efferent, p. 310

Select the correct term

9. B, p. 312
10. C, p. 312
11. C, p. 312
12. A, p. 311
13. C, p. 312
14. A, p. 311
15. A, p. 311

Matching

16. C, p. 312
17. A, p. 313
18. E, p. 313
19. B, p. 313
20. D, p. 313

Choose the term

21. C, p. 311
22. D, p. 311
23. E, p. 316
24. A, p. 314
25. H, p. 314
26. B, p. 314
27. I, p. 314
28. F, p. 315
29. J, p. 316
30. G, p. 316

Circle the one that does *not* belong

31. Allergy (all others refer to antibodies)
32. Complement (all others refer to antigens)
33. Antigen (all others refer to monoclonal antibodies)
34. Complement (all others refer to allergy)
35. Monoclonal (all others refer to complement)

Circle the correct answer

36. D, p. 317
37. D, p. 320
38. C, p. 320
39. B, p. 310
40. C, p. 318
41. C, p. 318
42. E, p. 321
43. E, p. 321
44. C, p. 321
45. E, p. 321
46. E, p. 321
47. D, p. 319
48. E, p. 319
49. A, p. 321
50. B, p. 322

Fill in the blanks

51. Stem cell, p. 317
52. Activated B cell, p. 320
53. Plasma cells, p. 321
54. Thymus gland, p. 321
55. Azidothymidine or AZT, p. 319
56. AIDS, p. 319
57. Vaccine, p. 319

Unscramble the words

58. Complement
59. Immunity
60. Clones
61. Interferon
62. Memory cells

Applying what you know

63. Interferon may possibly decrease the severity of the chickenpox virus.
64. AIDS
65. Baby Phelps had no means of producing T cells, thus making him susceptible to several diseases. Placing him in isolation was a means of controlling his exposure to these diseases.
66. WORD FIND

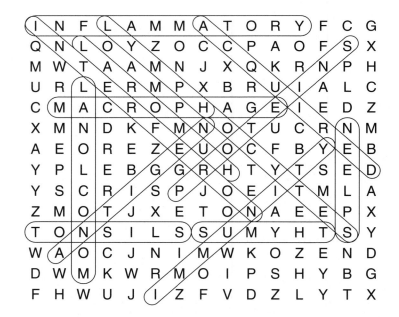

Crossword puzzle

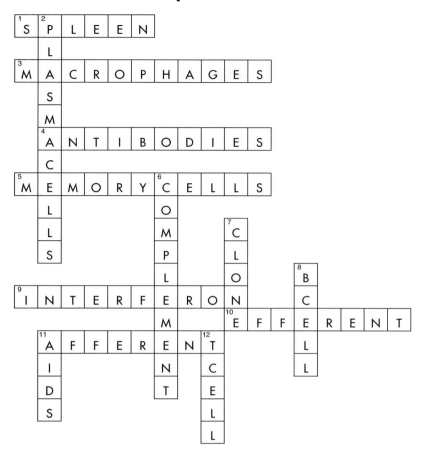

Check your knowledge

MULTIPLE CHOICE

1. A, p. 321
2. A, p. 308
3. D, p. 319
4. B, p. 319
5. D, p. 317
6. B, p. 316
7. D, p. 316
8. A, p. 317
9. D, p. 316
10. C, p. 314

MATCHING

11. E, p. 312
12. D, p. 321
13. I, p. 318
14. H, p. 319
15. G, p. 316
16. B, p. 309
17. A, p. 309
18. J, p. 322
19. C, p. 314
20. F, p. 314

B CELL DEVELOPMENT

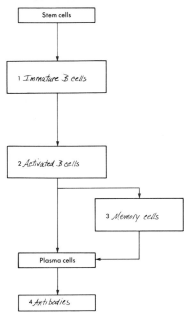

1. Immature B cells
2. Activated B cells
3. Memory cells
4. Antibodies

PRINCIPAL ORGANS OF LYMPHATIC SYSTEM

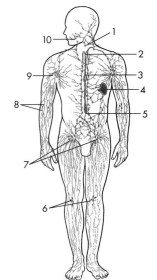

1. Cervical lymph nodes
2. Thymus
3. Thoracic duct
4. Spleen
5. Cisterna chyli
6. Popliteal lymph nodes
7. Inguinal lymph nodes
8. Lymph vessels
9. Axillary lymph nodes
10. Submandibular nodes

FUNCTION OF SENSITIZED T CELLS

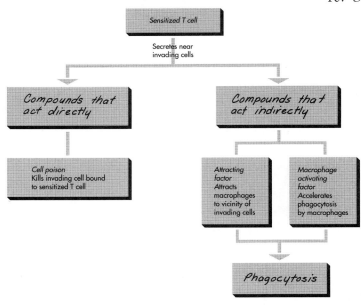

CHAPTER 13
THE RESPIRATORY SYSTEM

Matching

1. J, p. 331
2. G, p. 332
3. A, p. 332
4. I, p. 335
5. B, p. 335
6. F, p. 332
7. C, p. 332
8. H, p. 332
9. D, p. 332
10. E, p. 331

Fill in the blanks

11. Air distributor, p. 331
12. Gas exchanger, p. 331
13. Filters, p. 332
14. Warms, p. 332
15. Humidifies, p. 332
16. Nose, p. 332
17. Pharynx, p. 332
18. Larynx, p. 332
19. Trachea, p. 332
20. Bronchi, p. 332
21. Lungs, p. 332
22. Alveoli, p. 332
23. Diffusion, p. 332
24. Respiratory membrane, p. 332
25. Surface, p. 332

Circle the one that does *not* belong

26. Oropharynx (all others refer to the nose)
27. Conchae (all others refer to paranasal sinuses)
28. Epiglottis (all others refer to the pharynx)
29. Uvula (all others refer to the adenoids)
30. Larynx (all others refer to the eustachian tubes)
31. Tonsils (all others refer to the larynx)
32. Eustachian tube (all others refer to the tonsils)
33. Pharynx (all others refer to the larynx)

Select the correct term

34. A, p. 335
35. B, p. 338
36. A, p. 335
37. A, p. 336
38. A, p. 335
39. B, p. 338
40. B, p. 338
41. C, p. 338

Fill in the blanks

42. Trachea, p. 338
43. Cartilage (C-rings), p. 339
44. Heimlich maneuver, pp. 339 and 341
45. Primary bronchi, p. 340
46. Alveolar sacs, p. 340
47. Apex, p. 342
48. Pleura, p. 342
49. Pleurisy, p. 344
50. Pneumothorax, p. 344

True or false

51. Breathing, p. 346
52. Expiration, p. 347
53. Down, p. 346 (Review Chapter 2)
54. Internal, p. 347
55. T
56. 1 pint, p. 349
57. T
58. Vital capacity, p. 349
59. T

Circle the best answer

60. E, p. 346
61. C, p. 347
62. C, p. 347
63. B, p. 346
64. D, p. 349
65. D, p. 349
66. D, p. 349

Matching

67. E, p. 351
68. B, p. 351
69. G, p. 351
70. A, p. 351
71. F, p. 351
72. D, p. 351
73. C, p. 351

Unscramble the words

74. Pleurisy
75. Bronchitis
76. Epistaxis
77. Adenoids
78. Inspiration

Applying what you know

79. During the day Mr. Gorski's cilia are paralyzed because of his heavy smoking. They use the time, when Mr. Gorski is asleep, to sweep accumulations of mucus and bacteria toward the pharynx. When he awakes, these collections are waiting to be eliminated.
80. Swelling of the tonsils or adenoids caused by infection may make it difficult or impossible for air to travel from the nose into the throat. The individual may be forced to breathe through the mouth.

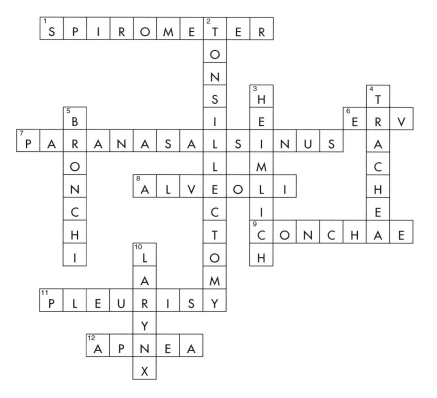

Crossword puzzle

Check your knowledge

MULTIPLE CHOICE

1. A, p. 351
2. B, p. 338
3. D, p. 342
4. B, p. 349
5. A, p. 342
6. D, p. 338
7. A, p. 339
8. C, p. 346
9. D, p. 346
10. B, p. 338

MATCHING

11. E, p. 338
12. I, p. 346
13. A, p. 342
14. G, p. 344
15. D, p. 345
16. B, p. 338
17. C, p. 335
18. H, p. 338
19. F, p. 347
20. J, p. 342

SAGITTAL VIEW OF FACE AND NECK

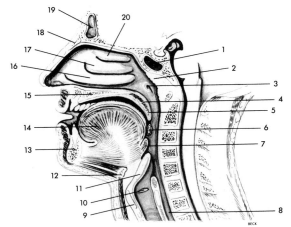

1. Sphenoid air sinus
2. Pharyngeal tonsil (adenoids)
3. Auditory tube
4. Soft palate
5. Uvula
6. Palatine tonsil
7. Lingual tonsil
8. Esophagus
9. Thyroid cartilage
10. Vocal cords
11. Epiglottis
12. Hyoid bone
13. Mandible
14. Tongue
15. Hard palate
16. Inferior concha
17. Middle concha
18. Nasal bone
19. Frontal air sinus
20. Superior concha

RESPIRATORY ORGANS

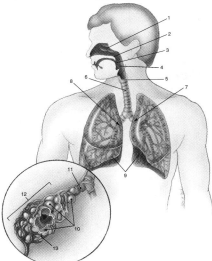

1. Nasal cavity
2. Nasopharynx
3. Oropharynx
4. Laryngopharynx
5. Larynx
6. Trachea
7. Left primary bronchus
8. Right primary bronchus
9. Bronchioles
10. Alveoli
11. Alveolar duct
12. Alveolar sac
13. Capillary

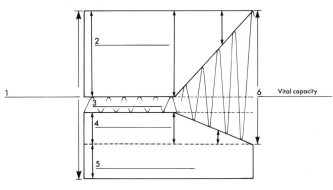

PULMONARY VENTILATION VOLUMES

1. Total lung capacity
2. Inspiratory reserve volume
3. Tidal volume
4. Expiratory reserve volume
5. Residual volume

CHAPTER 14
THE DIGESTIVE SYSTEM

Fill in the blanks

1. Gastrointestinal tract or G.I. tract, p. 361
2. Mechanical, p. 361
3. Chemical, p. 361
4. Feces, p. 362
5. Digestion, absorption, metabolism, p. 362
6. Parietal peritoneum, p. 363
7. Mouth, anus, p. 362
8. Lumen, p. 362
9. Mucosa, p. 362
10. Submucosa, p. 362
11. Peristalsis, p. 363
12. Serosa, p. 363
13. Mesentery, p. 363

Select the correct term

14. A, p. 362
15. B, p. 362
16. B, p. 362
17. A, p. 362
18. A, p. 362
19. A, p. 362
20. A, p. 362
21. A, p. 362
22. B, p. 362
23. B, p. 362
24. B, p. 362
25. B, p. 362

Circle the best answer

26. E, p. 364
27. C, p. 365
28. E, p. 366
29. D, p. 367
30. B, p. 367
31. C, p. 366
32. D, p. 366
33. D, p. 366
34. D, p. 368
35. A, p. 368
36. C, p. 368
37. A, p. 368
38. A, p. 366
39. B, p. 366
40. C, p. 366

Fill in the blanks

41. Pharynx, p. 368
42. Esophagus, p. 368
43. Stomach, p. 368
44. Cardiac sphincter, p. 369
45. Chyme, p. 370
46. Fundus, p. 370
47. Body, p. 370
48. Pylorus, p. 370
49. Pyloric sphincter, p. 370
50. Small intestine, p. 371

Matching

51. D, p. 370
52. J, p. 371
53. G, p. 371
54. A, p. 368
55. H, p. 371
56. B, p. 370
57. C, p. 370
58. E, p. 373
59. I, p. 371
60. F, p. 371

Circle the best answer

61. C, p. 371
62. B, pp. 370 and 371
63. A, p. 373
64. A, p. 374
65. B, p. 371
66. E, p. 373
67. D, p. 373
68. D, p. 373 (Review Chapter 9; hormones circulate in blood)
69. B, p. 374
70. C, p. 373

True or false

71. Vitamin K, p. 376
72. No villi are present in the large intestine, p. 376
73. Diarrhea, p. 377
74. Cecum, p. 378
75. Hepatic, p. 378
76. Sigmoid, p. 378
77. T
78. T
79. Parietal, p. 378
80. Mesentery, p. 379

Multiple choice

81. B, p. 380
82. D, p. 380
83. C, p. 380
84. C, p. 380
85. C, p. 380

86. Fill in the blank areas on the chart below.

CHEMICAL DIGESTION

DIGESTIVE JUICES AND ENZYMES	SUBSTANCE DIGESTED (OR HYDROLYZED)	RESULTING PRODUCT
Saliva	1. Starch (polysaccharide)	
Gastric Juice		2. Partially digested proteins
Pancreatic Juice		3. Starch, peptides, and amino acids
	4. Fats emulsified by bile	
	5. Starch	
Intestinal Juice	6. Peptides	
7. Sucrase	8. Lactose	
		9. Glucose

Unscramble the words

87. Bolus
88. Chyme
89. Papilla
90. Peritoneum
91. Lace apron

Applying what you know

92. Ulcer
93. Pylorospasm
94. Basal metabolic rate or protein-bound iodine to determine thyroid function

95. WORD FIND

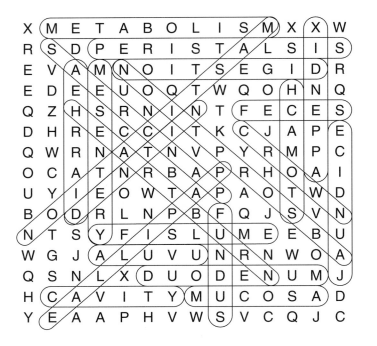

```
X M E T A B O L I S M X X W
R S D P E R I S T A L S I S
E V A M N O I T S E G I D R
E D E E U O Q T W Q O H N Q
Q Z H S R N I N T F E C E S
D H R E C C I T K C J A P E
Q W R N A T N V P Y R M P C
O C A T N R B A P R H O A I
U Y I E O W T A P A O T W D
B O D R L N P B F Q J S V N
N T S Y F I S L U M E E B U
W G J A L U V U N R N W O A
Q S N L X D U O D E N U M J
H C A V I T Y M U C O S A D
Y E A A P H V W S V C Q J C
```

Crossword puzzle

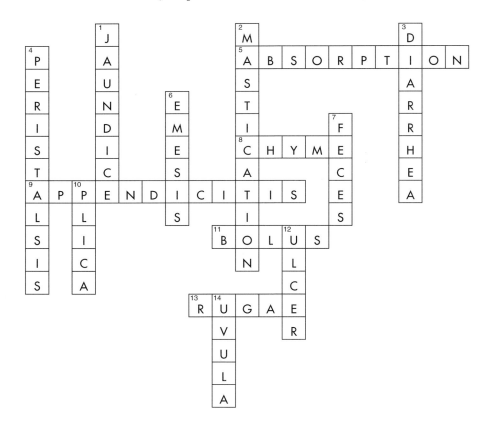

Check your knowledge

MULTIPLE CHOICE

1. A, p. 374
2. C, p. 370
3. A, p. 371
4. B, p. 367
5. B, p. 363
6. B, p. 371
7. B, p. 379
8. C, p. 380
9. C, p. 380
10. A, p. 380

COMPLETION

11. N, p. 378
12. J, p. 379
13. P, p. 380
14. Q, R, A, p. 371
15. W, p. 373
16. H, K, D, p. 362
17. E, p. 374
18. T, U, C, X, p. 362
19. G, p. 369
20. I, O, S, F, p. 366

DIGESTIVE ORGANS

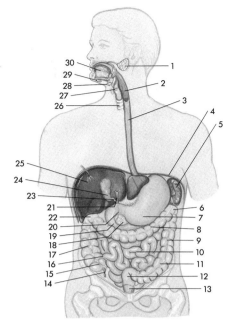

1. Parotid gland
2. Pharynx
3. Esophagus
4. Diaphragm
5. Spleen
6. Splenic flexure
7. Stomach
8. Transverse colon
9. Descending colon
10. Ileum
11. Sigmoid colon
12. Rectum
13. Anal canal
14. Vermiform appendix
15. Cecum
16. Ileocecal valve
17. Ascending colon
18. Pancreas
19. Duodenum
20. Common bile duct
21. Hepatic bile duct
22. Hepatic flexure
23. Cystic duct
24. Gallbladder
25. Liver
26. Trachea
27. Larynx
28. Submandibular gland
29. Sublingual gland
30. Tongue

TOOTH

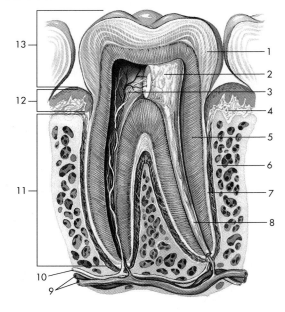

1. Enamel
2. Pulp
3. Pulp cavity
4. Gingiva (gum)
5. Dentin
6. Periodontal membrane
7. Cementum
8. Root canal
9. Vein and artery
10. Nerve
11. Root
12. Neck
13. Crown

THE SALIVARY GLANDS

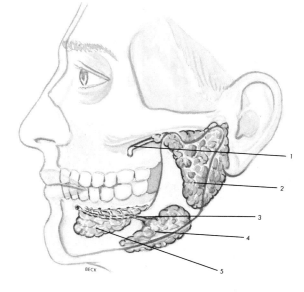

1. Parotid duct
2. Parotid gland
3. Submandibular duct
4. Submandibular gland
5. Sublingual gland

332   Answer Key

STOMACH

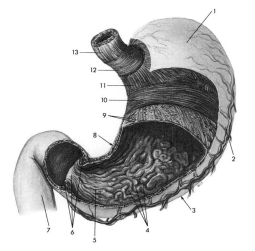

GALLBLADDER AND BILE DUCTS

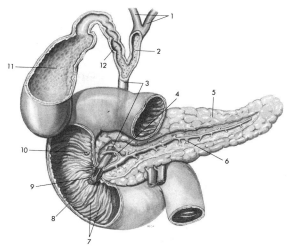

1. Fundus
2. Body
3. Greater curvature
4. Rugae
5. Pylorus
6. Pyloric sphincter
7. Duodenum
8. Lesser curvature
9. Oblique muscle layer
10. Circular muscle layer
11. Longitudinal muscle
12. Cardiac sphincter
13. Esophagus

1. Right and left hepatic ducts
2. Common hepatic duct
3. Common bile duct
4. Accessory duct
5. Pancreas
6. Pancreatic duct
7. Duodenum
8. Major duodenal papilla
9. Sphincter muscles
10. Minor duodenal papilla
11. Gallbladder
12. Cystic duct

THE SMALL INTESTINE

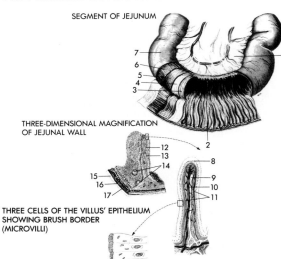

SEGMENT OF JEJUNUM

THREE-DIMENSIONAL MAGNIFICATION
OF JEJUNAL WALL

THREE CELLS OF THE VILLUS' EPITHELIUM
SHOWING BRUSH BORDER
(MICROVILLI)

1. Mesentery
2. Plica
3. Mucosa
4. Submucosa
5. Circular muscle
6. Longitudinal muscle
7. Serosa
8. Epithelium of villus
9. Lacteal
10. Artery
11. Vein
12. Plica
13. Submucosa
14. Lymph nodules
15. Serosa
16. Circular muscle
17. Longitudinal muscle

THE LARGE INTESTINE

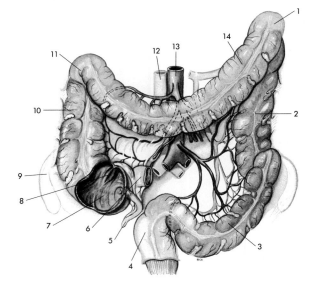

1. Splenic flexure
2. Descending colon
3. Sigmoid colon
4. Rectum
5. Vermiform appendix
6. Ileum
7. Cecum
8. Ileocecal valve
9. Ilium
10. Ascending colon
11. Hepatic flexure
12. Inferior vena cava
13. Aorta
14. Transverse colon

CHAPTER 15
NUTRITION AND
METABOLISM

Fill in the blanks

1. Bile, p. 390
2. Prothrombin, p. 390
3. Fibrinogen, p. 390
4. Iron, p. 390
5. Hepatic portal vein, p. 390

Matching

6. B, p. 392
7. A, p. 390
8. C, p. 393
9. D, p. 394
10. E, p. 394
11. A, p. 390
12. E, p. 394
13. A, p. 390

Circle the one that does *not* belong

14. Bile (all others refer to carbohydrate metabolism)
15. Amino acids (all others refer to fat metabolism)
16. M (All other refer to vitamins)
17. Iron (all others refer to protein metabolism)

18. Insulin (all others tend to increase blood glucose)
19. Folic acid (all others are minerals)
20. Ascorbic acid (all others refer to the B-complex vitamins)

Circle the correct answer

21. C, p. 394
22. A, p. 397
23. C, p. 397
24. B, p. 398
25. B, p. 398
26. A, p. 398
27. C, p. 398
28. D, p. 398
29. A, p. 397

Unscramble the words

30. Liver
31. Catabolism
32. Amino
33. Pyruvic
34. Evaporation

Applying what you know

35. Weight loss; Anorexia nervosa
36. Iron; Meat, eggs, vegetables and legumes
37. He was carbohydrate loading (also called glycogen loading), which allows the muscles to sustain aerobic exercise for up to 50% longer than usual.

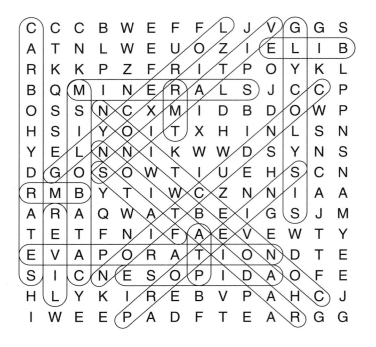

Crossword puzzle

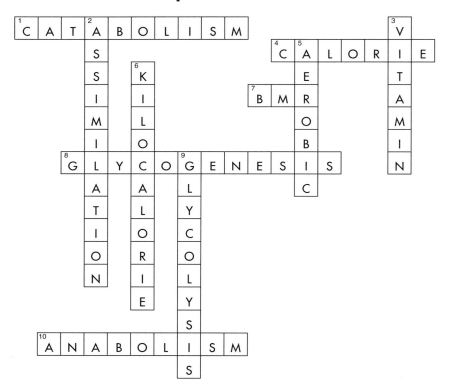

Check your knowledge

MULTIPLE CHOICE

1. B, p. 389
2. A, p. 390
3. C, p. 392
4. C, p. 397
5. B, p. 397
6. B, p. 392
7. A, p. 392
8. A, p. 398
9. B, p. 390
10. D, p. 390

COMPLETION

11. C, D, I, p. 389
12. E, p. 391
13. J, p. 391
14. G, p. 390
15. B, p. 392
16. D, p. 392
17. L, p. 393
18. A, p. 394
19. K, H, p. 394
20. F, p. 390

CHAPTER 16 URINARY SYSTEM

Circle the correct answer

1. E, p. 405
2. C, p. 405
3. E, p. 405
4. C, p. 406
5. E, p. 410
6. C, p. 409
7. B. p. 410
8. E, p. 410
9. C, p. 410
10. C, p. 410
11. B, p. 411 (Review Chapter 9)
12. D, p. 411

Choose the correct term

13. G, p. 405
14. I, p. 412
15. H, p. 403
16. B, p. 405
17. K, p. 405
18. F, p. 405
19. J, p. 405
20. D, p. 405
21. L, p. 406
22. C, p. 405
23. M, p. 413
24. A, p. 405

Indicate which organ is identified

25. B, p. 414
26. C, p. 414
27. A, p. 412
28. B, p. 412
29. C, p. 415
30. C, p. 415
31. A, p. 412
32. C, p. 414
33. B, p. 412
34. A, p. 412
35. B, p. 414

Fill in the blanks

36. Renal colic, p. 414
37. Mucous membrane, p. 412
38. Renal calculi, p. 416
39. Ultrasound, p. 416
40. Catheterization, p. 415
41. Renal pelvis, p. 412
42. Semen, p. 415
43. Urinary meatus, p. 414

Fill in the blanks

44. Micturition, p. 415
45. Urination, p. 415
46. Voiding, p. 415
47. Internal urethral, p. 415
48. Exit, p. 415
49. Urethra, p. 415
50. Voluntary, p. 415
51. Emptying reflex, p. 415
52. Urethra, p. 415
53. Retention, p. 415
54. Suppression, p. 416
55. Automatic bladder, p. 416

Unscramble the words

56. Calyx
57. Voiding
58. Papilla
59. Glomerulus
60. Pyramids

Applying what you know

61. Polyuria
62. Residual urine is often the cause of repeated cystitis.
63. A high percentage of catheterized patients develop cystitis, often due to poor aseptic technique when inserting the catheter.
64. WORD FIND

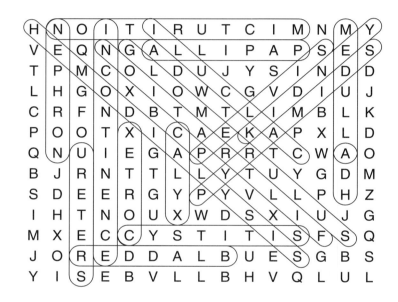

Crossword puzzle

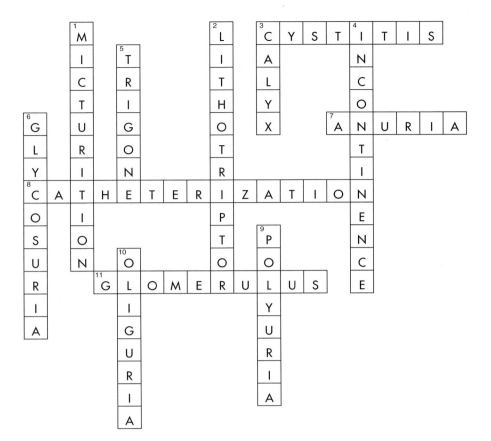

Check your knowledge

MULTIPLE CHOICE

1. D, p. 415
2. B, p. 413
3. D, p. 403
4. A, p. 411
5. C, p. 415
6. C, p. 411
7. B, p. 415
8. C, p. 412
9. B, p. 405
10. A, p. 405

MATCHING

11. E, p. 415
12. C, p. 412
13. F, p. 416
14. D, p. 415
15. J, p. 412
16. H, p. 412
17. A, p. 416
18. G, p. 412
19. I, p. 415
20. B, p. 411

URINARY SYSTEM

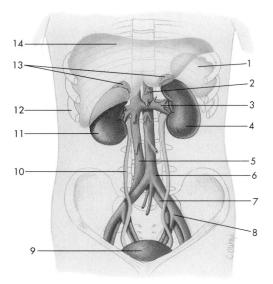

KIDNEY

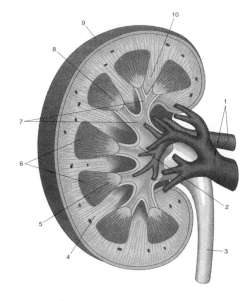

1. Spleen
2. Renal artery
3. Renal vein
4. Kidney (left)
5. Inferior vena cava
6. Abdominal aorta
7. Common iliac vein
8. Common iliac artery
9. Urinary bladder
10. Ureter
11. Kidney (right)
12. Tenth rib
13. Adrenal glands
14. Liver

1. Renal artery and vein
2. Pelvis
3. Ureter
4. Cortex
5. Pyramid
6. Medulla
7. Calyx
8. Papilla
9. Fibrous capsule
10. Renal column

NEPHRON

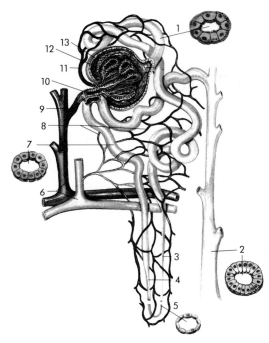

1. Proximal convoluted tubule
2. Collecting tubule
3. Descending limb of Henle's loop
4. Ascending limb of Henle's loop
5. Segment of Henle's loop
6. Artery and vein
7. Distal convoluted tubule
8. Peritubular capillaries
9. Afferent arteriole
10. Juxtaglomerular apparatus
11. Efferent arteriole
12. Glomerulus
13. Bowman's capsule

CHAPTER 17
FLUID AND ELECTROLYTE BALANCE

Circle the correct answer

1. Inside, p. 424
2. Extracellular, p. 424
3. Extracellular, p. 424
4. Lower, p. 424
5. More, p. 424
6. Decline, p. 425
7. Less, p. 425
8. Decreases, p. 425
9. 55%, p. 424
10. "Fluid balance," p. 424

Circle the correct answer

11. A, p. 428
12. D, p. 428
13. A, p. 428
14. A, p. 428
15. C, p. 428
16. E, p. 427
17. D, p. 426
18. D, p. 426
19. C, p. 430
20. B, p. 428
21. D, p. 429
22. E, p. 431
23. B, p. 432
24. B, p. 432
25. B, p. 432
26. E, p. 429

True or false

27. Catabolism, p. 425
28. T
29. T
30. Nonelectrolyte, p. 427
31. T
32. Hypervolemia, p. 430
33. Tubular function, p. 429
34. 2400 ml, p. 427
35. T
36. 100 mEq, p. 429

Fill in the blanks

37. Dehydration, p. 432
38. Decreases, p. 432
39. Decrease, p. 432
40. Overhydration, p. 432
41. Intravenous fluids, p. 432
42. Heart, p. 432

Applying what you know

43. Ms. Titus could not accurately measure water intake created by foods or catabolism, nor could she measure output created by lungs, skin, or the intestines.
44. A careful record of fluid intake and output should be maintained and the patient should be monitored for signs and symptoms of electrolyte and water imbalance.
45. WORD FIND

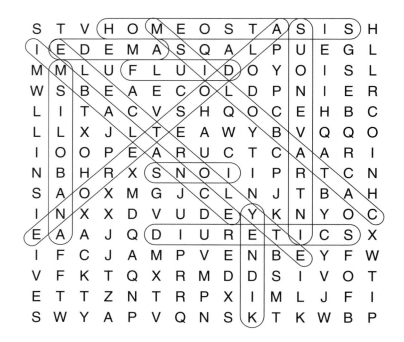

Crossword puzzle

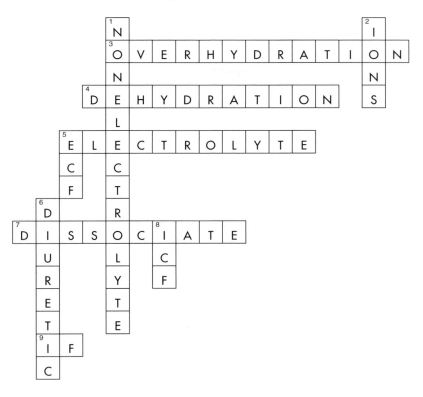

Check your knowledge

MULTIPLE CHOICE

1. A, p. 424
2. D, p. 427
3. D, p. 432
4. C, p. 432
5. A, p. 430
6. B, p. 428
7. D, p. 427
8. A, p. 429
9. A, p. 428
10. D, p. 428

COMPLETION

11. E, p. 429
12. B, p. 429
13. J, M, K, p. 424
14. F, p. 427
15. D, p. 428
16. L, p. 427
17. I, p. 432
18. C, p. 432
19. H, A, p. 426
20. N, p. 423

CHAPTER 18
ACID-BASE BALANCE

Choose the correct term
1. B, p. 438
2. A, p. 438
3. A, p. 438
4. B, p. 438
5. B, p. 438
6. B, p. 438
7. B, p. 438
8. A, p. 438
9. B, p. 438
10. B, p. 438

Circle the correct answer
11. E, p. 439
12. E, p. 439
13. A, p. 439
14. E, p. 440
15. C, p. 440
16. D, p. 440
17. C, p. 442
18. B, p. 443
19. D, p. 443
20. E, p. 443
21. E, p. 443

True or false
22. Buffer (instead of heart), p. 438
23. Buffer pairs, p. 439
24. T
25. T
26. Alkalosis, p. 442
27. Kidneys, p. 442
28. T
29. Kidneys, p. 444
30. Lungs, p. 444

Write the letter of the correct term
31. E, p. 445
32. G, p. 446
33. F, p. 445
34. A, p. 445
35. I, p. 446
36. B, p. 445
37. H, p. 445
38. C, p. 445
39. D, p. 445
40. J, p. 445

Applying what you know
41. Normal saline contains chloride ions which replace bicarbonate ions and thus relieve the bicarbonate excess that occurs during severe vomiting.
42. Most citrus fruits, although acid-tasting, are fully oxidized during metabolism and have little effect on acid-base balance. Cranberry juice is one of the few exceptions.
43. Milk of magnesia, because it is base. Milk is slightly acidic. (See chart, p. 438)

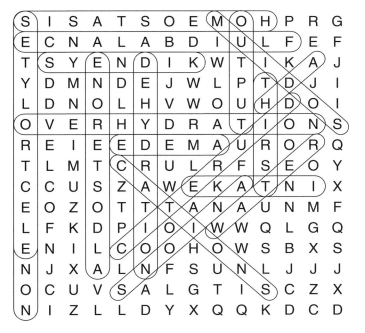

Crossword puzzle

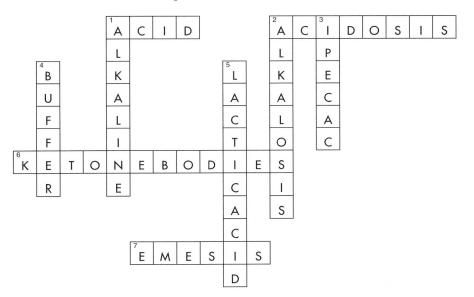

Check your knowledge

MULTIPLE CHOICE

1. A, p. 439
2. C, p. 439
3. A, p. 442
4. D, p. 438
5. A, p. 446
6. D, p. 445

7. D, p. 439
8. D, p. 445
9. D, p. 439
10. A, p. 440

11. G, p. 438
12. C, p. 437
13. I, p. 439
14. E, p. 442
15. F, p. 442
16. A, p. 445
17. B, p. 445
18. D, p. 439
19. J, p. 442
20. H, p. 446

CHAPTER 19
THE REPRODUCTIVE SYSTEMS

Matching

1. D, p. 454
2. C, p. 454
3. E, p. 453
4. B, p. 454
5. A, p. 453
6. C, p. 454
7. A, p. 454
8. D, p. 453
9. B, p. 454
10. E, p. 454

Circle the correct answer

11. B, p. 455
12. C, p. 455
13. A, p. 455
14. D, p. 458
15. E, p. 455
16. D, p. 458
17. C, p. 459
18. C, p. 456
19. A, p. 458
20. B, p. 458

Fill in the blanks

21. Testes, p. 455
22. Spermatozoa or sperm, p. 456
23. Ovum, p. 454
24. Testosterone, p. 459
25. Interstitial cells, p. 459
26. Masculinizing, p. 459
27. Anabolic, p. 459

Choose the correct term

28. B, p. 460
29. H, p. 462
30. G, p. 460
31. A, p. 460
32. F, p. 460
33. C, p. 460
34. I, p. 460
35. E, p. 460
36. D, p. 461
37. J, p. 460

Matching

38. D, p. 462
39. C, p. 462
40. B, p. 462
41. A, p. 462
42. E, p. 462

Select the correct term

43. A, p. 467
44. B, p. 466
45. A, p. 467
46. B, p. 465
47. A, p. 467
48. A, p. 467
49. A, p. 467
50. B, p. 462

Fill in the blanks

51. Gonads, p. 462
52. Oogenesis, p. 463
53. Meiosis, p. 463
54. half or 23, p. 464
55. Fertilization, p. 464
56. 46, p. 464
57. Estrogen, p. 464
58. Progesterone, p. 464
59. Secondary sexual characteristics, p. 464
60. Menstrual cycle, p. 464
61. Puberty, p. 465

Select the correct term

62. A, p. 466
63. B, p. 466
64. C, p. 466
65. B, p. 466
66. A, p. 465, and C, p. 466
67. B, p. 466
68. A, p. 465
69. A, p. 465
70. C, p. 466
71. B, p. 471

Matching

72. D, p. 466
73. E. p. 467
74. B, p. 467
75. C, p. 467
76. A, p. 467
77. E, p. 467
78. A, p. 467
79. D, p. 467
80. B, p. 468
81. C, p. 468

True or false

82. "Menarche," p. 468
83. One, p. 471
84. 14, p. 471
85. The menstrual period, p. 471
86. T, p. 471
87. Anterior, p. 471

Write the letter of the correct hormone

88. B, p. 471
89. A, p. 471
90. B, p. 471
91. B, p. 471
92. A, p. 471

Applying what you know

93. Yes. The testes are not only essential organs of reproduction, but they are also responsible for the "masculinizing" hormone. Without this hormone, Mr. Belinki will have no desire to reproduce.

94. He may be sterile. His sperm count may be too low to allow for reproduction, but the remaining testicle will produce enough masculinizing hormone to prevent impotency.

95. The uterine tubes are not attached to the ovaries and infections can exit at this area and enter the abdominal cavity.

96. Yes it is. Yes she will. Without the hormones from the ovaries to initiate the menstrual cycle, Mrs. Harlan will no longer have a menstrual cycle and can be considered to be in menopause (cessation of menstrual cycle).

97. No. Delceta will still have her ovaries, which are the source of her hormones, so she will not experience menopause due to this procedure.

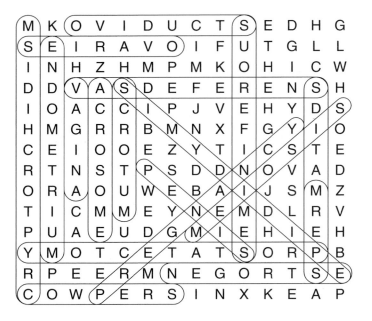

Crossword puzzle

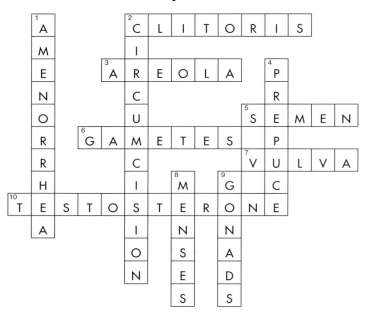

Check your knowledge

MULTIPLE CHOICE

1. A, p. 467
2. D, p. 470
3. D, p. 460
4. C, p. 458
5. C, p. 462

6. A, p. 454
7. B, p. 455
8. C, p. 461
9. A, p. 467
10. D, p. 470

COMPLETION

11. C, p. 466
12. L, p. 455
13. H, p. 460
14. G, p. 471
15. F, p. 460
16. K, p. 461
17. B, p. 466
18. D, p. 464
19. J, p. 471
20. I, p. 471

MALE REPRODUCTIVE ORGANS

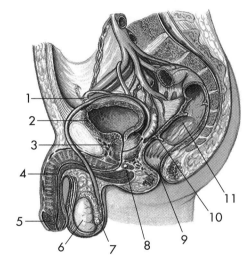

1. Ductus deferens
2. Bladder
3. Prostate gland
4. Urethra
5. Penis
6. Testis
7. Epididymis
8. Bulbourethral gland
9. Anus
10. Seminal vesicle
11. Rectum

TUBULES OF TESTIS AND EPIDIDYMIS

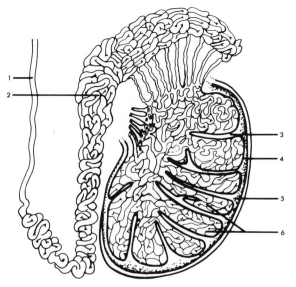

1. Ductus (vas) deferens
2. Body of epididymis
3. Septum
4. Lobule
5. Tunica albuginea
6. Seminiferous tubules

VULVA

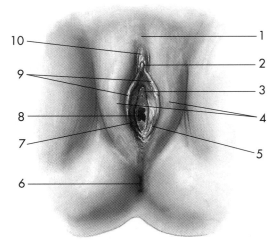

1. Mons pubis
2. Clitoris
3. Orifice of urethra
4. Labia majora
5. Opening of greater vestibular gland
6. Anus
7. Vestibule
8. Orifice of vagina
9. Labia minora
10. Prepuce

BREAST

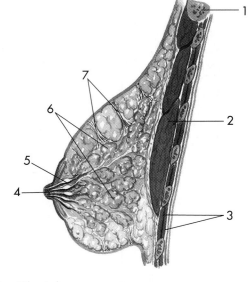

1. Clavicle
2. Pectoralis major muscle
3. Intercostal muscles
4. Nipple
5. Lactiferous duct
6. Alveoli
7. Suspensory ligaments of Cooper

FEMALE PELVIS

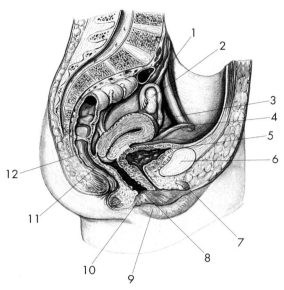

1. Fallopian tube (uterine)
2. Ovary
3. Uterus
4. Fundus of uterus
5. Urinary bladder
6. Symphysis pubis
7. Clitoris
8. Vagina
9. Labium majus
10. Labium minus
11. Cervix
12. Rectum

UTERUS AND ADJACENT STRUCTURES

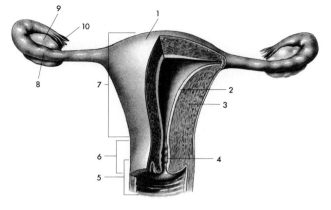

1. Fundus
2. Endometrium
3. Myometrium
4. Cervical canal
5. Vagina
6. Cervix
7. Body
8. Uterine (Fallopian) tube
9. Ovary
10. Fimbriae

CHAPTER 20
GROWTH AND
DEVELOPMENT

Fill in the blanks

1. Conception, p. 482
2. Birth, p. 482
3. Embryology, p. 482
4. Oviduct, p. 482
5. Zygote, p. 483
6. Morula, p. 483
7. Blastocyst, p. 483
8. Amniotic cavity, p. 484
9. Chorion, p. 484
10. Placenta, p. 484

Choose the correct term

11. G, p. 485
12. F, p. 487
13. C, p. 491
14. B, p. 486
15. A, p. 485
16. H, p. 489
17. E, p. 489
18. D, p. 487
19. I, p. 487
20. J, p. 491

Circle the correct answer

21. E, p. 492
22. E, p. 492
23. E, p. 493
24. A, p. 493
25. B, p. 493
26. C, p. 493
27. B, p. 493
28. D, p. 494
29. E, p. 494
30. D, p. 494
31. A, p. 494
32. C, p. 494
33. C, p. 495
34. C, p. 494
35. E, p. 494

Write the letter of the correct word

36. F, p. 491
37. A, p. 492
38. C, p. 494
39. H, p. 494

40. D, p. 494
41. B, p. 492
42. E, p. 494
43. G, p. 492
44. I, p. 495

Fill in the blanks

45. Lipping, p. 495
46. Osteoarthritis, p. 495
47. Nephron, p. 495
48. Barrel chest, p. 495
49. Atherosclerosis, p. 497
50. Arteriosclerosis, p. 497
51. Hypertension, p. 497
52. Presbyopia, p. 497
53. Cataract, p. 497
54. Glaucoma, p. 497

Unscramble the words

55. Infancy
56. Postnatal
57. Organogenesis
58. Zygote
59. Childhood
60. Fertilization

Applying what you know

61. Normal
62. Only about 40% of the taste buds present at age 30 remain at age 75.
63. A significant loss of hair cells in the Organ of Corti causes a serious decline in the ability to hear certain frequencies.

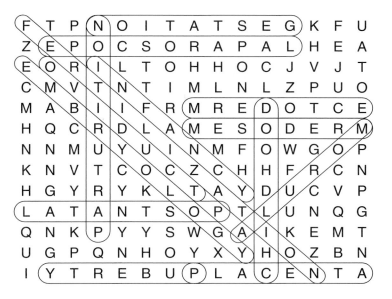

Crossword puzzle

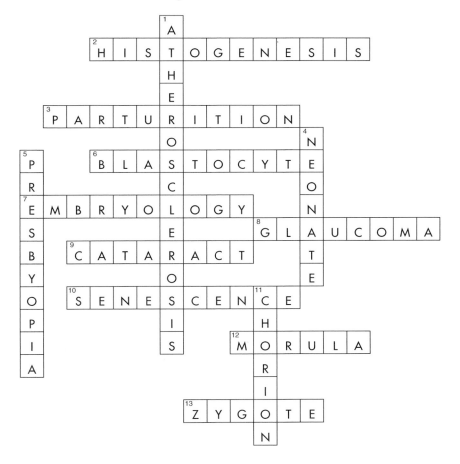

Check your knowledge

MULTIPLE CHOICE

1. C, p. 483
2. D, p. 495
3. D, p. 495
4. A, p. 492
5. D, p. 497
6. D, p. 497
7. C, p. 489
8. A, p. 495
9. C, p. 495
10. B, p. 489

MATCHING

11. E, p. 497
12. G, p. 497
13. C, p. 489
14. I, p. 497
15. H, p. 494
16. D, p. 484
17. J, p. 497
18. F, p. 495
19. A, p. 497
20. B, p. 484

FERTILIZATION AND IMPLANTATION

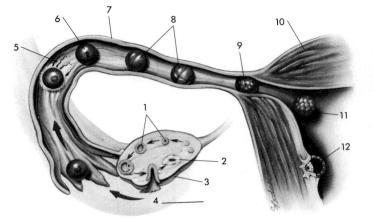

1. Developing follicles
2. Corpus luteum
3. Ovary
4. Ovulation
5. Spermatozoa (fertilization)
6. First mitosis
7. Uterine (Fallopian) tube
8. Divided zygote
9. Morula
10. Uterus
11. Blastocyst
12. Implantation